Public–Private Relations in Health Care

Public–Private Relations in Health Care

Justin Keen, Donald Light and Nicholas Mays

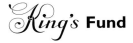

Published by
King's Fund Publishing
11–13 Cavendish Square
London W1G 0AN

ISBN 1 85717 257 4

A CIP catalogue record for this book is available from the British Library

Available from:

King's Fund Bookshop
11–13 Cavendish Square
London
W1G 0AN

Tel: 020 7307 2591
Fax: 020 7307 2801

Printed and bound in Great Britain by Henry Ling Ltd., Dorchester, Dorset

Typeset by Peter Powell Origination & Print Limited

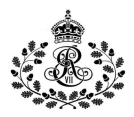

Contents

Acknowledgements

We are grateful to a number of people for their help in the research, writing and production of this book. We spoke to many people in the course of our research, and would particularly like to thank employees of the Association of British Insurers, Boots, BUPA, Federation of Dispensing Opticians, Financial Services Authority, General Healthcare Group, Insurance Ombudsman's Bureau, Legal and General, Norwich Union Healthcare, Nuffield Hospitals Group, PPP Healthcare, Research Council for Complementary Medicines, and Kate Thomas of the University of Sheffield.

We appreciate the help of H Maarse, K Okma, F Schut, and especially H Lieverdink, for their help with the Dutch section, and the generous help of Asling Byre and Desmond McCluskey on the Irish section of the book.

At the King's Fund, Kim Stirling provided able administrative support throughout. We are grateful to John Appleby, Michelle Dixon and Ian Wylie for their support during the production process. Thanks are also due to Trevor Anderson and Anita Jane Reid for their careful organisation and copy-editing of the text.

We are grateful to the following for permission to reproduce figures and tables: The Stationery Office (Figure 1.1, Figure 2.1, Tables 2.4, 2.6, 2.7, 2.8), Laing and Buisson (part of Table 2.2, Table 2.5), Institute of Employment Studies (Figure 2.3), Department of Health (Figure 2.4), HSA (Table 3.5), Joseph Rowntree Foundation (Figures 4.1 and 4.2) and the Competition Commission (Figure 4.5).

About the authors

Justin Keen is Professor of Health Politics and Information Management at the Nuffield Institute for Health at the University of Leeds. He is also Deputy Director of the Knowledge Management Centre at the School of Public Policy, University College London. He was Fellow in Health Systems at the King's Fund, 1998–2001.

Donald Light has been contributing international perspectives and in-depth reports to the NHS reforms since their inception in 1990. He is Professor of Comparative Health Care Systems at the University of Medicine and Dentistry of New Jersey, USA, and Fellow at the Wharton School of Management at the University of Pennsylvania.

Nicholas Mays is Principal Adviser in the Social Policy Branch of the New Zealand Treasury and Visiting Professor in the Department of Public Health and Policy at the London School of Hygiene and Tropical Medicine, University of London. Between January 1994 and September 1998, he was, successively, Director of Health Services Research and Director of the Health Systems Programme at the King's Fund.

Chapter 1

Introduction

Public–private relations

Health care is rarely out of the headlines in UK newspapers these days. There is a seemingly never-ending stream of stories about people who have received poor-quality treatment in the NHS. One story that received wide publicity occurred during the 2001 election campaign:

> Tony Blair's carefully orchestrated election tour was finally disrupted yesterday ... Sharron Storer, 38, from Hall Green, Birmingham, blocked his entrance to Queen Elizabeth Hospital in Edgbaston, Birmingham. She was distraught about the treatment of her partner, Keith Sedgwick, 48, who has cancer.[1]

There are also stories about people who have had bad experiences in private hospitals and clinics:

> When John came round from the second operation things obviously weren't as they should have been. He had low blood pressure and a high temperature ... [John said] I wouldn't use the private system for anything now. I feel frustrated with the system and terribly bitter.[2]

> The NHS is being forced to cancel operations because intensive-care beds are being taken up by private patients whose surgery has gone wrong ... Senior figures in the Intensive Care Society, which represents doctors working in Britain's 251 intensive care units, estimate the figure will soon rise above 1000 [per year] as more people use the private sector to avoid NHS waiting lists.[3]

In addition, there are stories comparing the two sectors. *The Express* reported the experiences of two sisters who had undergone the same surgical procedure:

> Penny was able to undergo surgery at the Park Hospital, Nottingham, two weeks [after an out-patient consultation] ... Katherine had her [NHS] operation in October after waiting five months.

Penny was quoted as saying:

> *We are identical twins who had operations to correct identical defects, yet my recovery rate and the level of pain I suffered in the aftermath of the operation was far better.*[4]

These stories are usually presented as being of 'human interest', but there have been a number of occasions in recent years when an individual case has become bound up in a political debate. The case of Keith Sedgwick is just one example. Such cases serve to crystallise important issues, such as the time people have to wait for treatment, and treatment quality and outcomes.

In most cases, the temperature of the debate slowly decreases, and health care carries on much as before. But since early 2000 the situation has changed. The Labour Government responded to media reports about poor-quality NHS services, and to a growing perception of under-funding of UK health care, by committing very substantial additional resources to the NHS for the years 2000–04. This will bring UK health spending closer to the European Union average, partially fulfilling a pledge made by Prime Minister Tony Blair early in the year.[5] At the same time, the Government departed from its long-standing policy of keeping private health care at arm's length from the NHS, with the Prime Minister stating that he had no ideological objection to closer relationships:

> *If you have a facility and you have the money, and just because it is private you do not use it – that is nonsensical.*[6]

In a number of statements made by Mr Blair[7] and health ministers,[8,9] it has become clear that the Government is committed to including private health care *provision* in its future plans. It appears to be ruling out a role for private *financing* of services, although it is still committed to private financing of capital projects, including hospital building and information technology investments.

This book investigates the nature and extent of private health care in the UK, the ways in which its fate is bound up with that of the NHS, and the extent to which the two sectors are regulated to achieve the best allocation of health care resources for 'UK plc'. We focus on final goods and services – on the financing and delivery of health care – and not on relationships between government, the NHS and industry. These production relationships are important in their own right, covering as they do the pharmaceutical industry, capital projects financed through the Private Finance Initiative (PFI), and research and development. The only reason for omitting them is that each one raises complex issues, distinct from those raised by financing and delivery of health care, and they merit detailed treatment elsewhere. In Chapter 1, we lay the ground for the rest of the book, setting out the overall structure of our arguments and outlining the historical context in which public–private relations have developed.

We think that there are three main reasons to write this book now. First, private health care is firmly on the UK policy agenda, and some of the policy prescriptions being floated involve an enhanced role for it in the future. Private sector thinking has become ever more prominent in public policy-making and practice over the last 20 years. From the early 1980s onwards, public services were popularly diagnosed as suffering from a number of deep-seated malaises – and the treatment being proposed was emulation of private sector practices. Almost all people working in the public services must now have experienced at least some of this treatment. The Labour Government has made clear its enthusiasm for some of the treatments prescribed. Indeed, we seem to be witnessing the blurring of the boundaries between the public and private realms.[10] Is this the right way to proceed in health care?

Second, the private health care sector, while substantially smaller than the NHS, is easily large enough to justify the attention of policy-makers. For example, the private medical insurance market is valued at around £2 billion each year, expenditure on over-the-counter medicines is around £2.5 billion, and we spend at least £450 million each year on leading complementary therapies. It is reasonable, therefore, to ask whether privately provided goods and services are safe and effective. The current government has begun its thinking and is beginning to frame policies, but there are many issues to be tackled.

Third, there are many significant public–private relationships in health care, typically deeply embedded in the structure of the UK health care system. Many NHS consultants maintain private practices alongside their NHS work. The NHS is an important purchaser of private acute elective services and is also one of the largest providers of these services. In some sectors of health care, there has been a shift from the provision of NHS services – such as continuing nursing care and dentistry – to private settings. The nature and boundaries of the NHS have changed, particularly over the last two decades, and may be set for further change in the future. Far from being marginal, these relationships are at the heart of the current health care debate. If the Government wishes to reduce NHS waiting times, for example, it may have to negotiate changes to the NHS consultants' contract, clarify the role of NHS pay beds (private beds in NHS hospitals), and understand how changes in the volume of surgery undertaken in the private sector will affect the volume undertaken in the NHS.

Principles and main issues

The main policy argument in this book is that the public–private relations embedded in the UK health care system at the founding of the NHS – such as consultants' rights to maintain private practices alongside NHS work – are still in place, but all of them must be reviewed. The scale of private activity has grown to the point where serious questions can be asked about the fairness or otherwise of the health care system as a whole, both public and private.

In pursuing our arguments in the course of the book, we ask three descriptive questions:

- What are the contours of the private sector, i.e. what work is done and how is it financed?
- What is the nature and extent of relationships between public and private health care?
- What arrangements are there for regulation of the public and private sectors, and of the interfaces between the two?

Then, in order to analyse our descriptive material, we employ a framework based on two general principles, equity and consumer protection, using them as judgement criteria for current and possible future policies. Both might appear to be straightforward, unexceptionable principles, and it is difficult to see why any policy-maker would consciously decide to make a health care system less fair, or expose patients to greater risks than are absolutely necessary. There are reasons to believe, however, that these two principles need more attention than they have received. The NHS Plan[11] contains a number of useful ideas about both equity and consumer protection. Yet the Plan marks the start of a debate, and processes of change, rather than the endpoint in a complex and politically difficult area.

Equity

In the financing and delivery of health care services, equity has centred largely on the principle that health care should be paid for, 'From each according to his ability, to each according to his need.' The World Health Report 2000 draws on the words of Aneurin Bevan, 'The essence of a satisfactory health service is that the rich and the poor are treated alike, that poverty is not a disability, and wealth is not advantaged.'[12] Specifically, the WHO measure of equitable financing is the ratio of total health care spending to total non-food spending per household. This concept of fairness echoes traditional European arguments for health care systems based on solidarity – those who are healthy and working contribute to the costs of medical services of those who are ill. The NHS was founded on this concept, which has led to it being financed progressively, through direct taxation.

The concept of social equity contrasts with that of actuarial equity, which is the basis for individually-tailored or risk-rated medical insurance.[13] Actuarial equity holds that people in the same class of risk and/or illness should contribute in proportion to the likely size and probability of their own health care costs. Thus, it would be unfair to make healthy adults pay for the health care costs of older people, or for the costs of younger people with diabetes or depression. Unhealthy people should pay for their own care costs. This ethic is the foundation of the US health care system, as we will see in Chapter 5, and around it has arisen an elaborate set of techniques for rating individuals' health risks. It is also the basis for voluntary private medical insurance in the UK.

Some countries, including the Republic of Ireland (which is discussed in Chapter 5), have modified the logic of actuarial fairness by requiring 'community-rating'. This means that all people who apply for private medical insurance are charged the same premium, regardless of risk. Some countries may also require guaranteed renewal of insurance policies every year, i.e. policies are annually renewable, so that an individual's current insurer must renew any current policy at the community rate, regardless of any change in the individual's health status during the contract year.

Given that countries have designed their health care systems according to different equity principles, we need to be clear which ones we are concerned with. A distinction is often made between horizontal and vertical equity:

- Horizontal equity: equal treatment for individuals who are equal in some respect. This implies equal shares of something. For example, everyone who needs a hip replacement should have one, having waited the same length of time, and the treatment should be of the same quality for all.

- Vertical equity: the proportionately unequal treatment of people who are unequal in some respect. People experience different illnesses, which require different resources to treat, in the course of their lives. Given that, generally speaking, people do not know how or when they will fall ill, and do not become ill deliberately, we might judge that it is appropriate to allocate resources on the basis of need for care. We therefore provide proportionately unequal treatment, with the proportions being based on an assessment of the resources needed for treatment.

In this book, we are interested in both horizontal and vertical equity. At present in the UK, people who need hip replacements and other surgical interventions do not have equal access to treatment. Some have to wait longer than others,[14] and the quality of care and treatment outcomes vary from place to place.[15] One of the private hospital sector's selling points is faster access to treatment, but this creates an important source of horizontal inequity within the UK system. It is therefore important to understand the extent to which the presence of the private sector leads to inequalities, and to think about what level of inequality – if any – society feels comfortable with.

Vertical equity is important because of the uneven distribution of illness and disability within society. The challenge is to decide on a basis for sharing out available health care resources between people with unequal needs. That is, we must consider what a fair or just distribution of resources for health care would actually be in practice.[16]

Our chosen approach is based on Rawls' celebrated theory of social justice,[17] which was applied to the assessment of health system reform in the USA by Daniels, Light and Caplan.[18] Rawls starts with the premise that people inevitably look after their own interests and advantages first. When people are asked the question, 'What kind of society would you be willing to live in if you were to start from behind a "veil of ignorance", where you do not know your position in society or how your life will turn out?', they tend to favour a society in which there is equality of opportunity to participate in life's experiences. This approach centres around providing fair equality of opportunity to participate in life's experiences.

Building on Rawls, Daniels *et al.* argue that it is acceptable for people to have unequal basic resources, as long as those with more resources do not use them to disadvantage the least well-off (his 'difference principle'). They then derived ten 'benchmarks of fairness' for health care policies (*see* Table 1.1) and criteria for assessing the fairness of a given practice or policy.

Table 1.1 Ten benchmarks of fairness*

Benchmark 1:	Universal Access – Coverage and Participation
Benchmark 2:	Universal Access – Minimising Non-financial Barriers
Benchmark 3:	Comprehensive and Uniform Benefits
Benchmark 4:	Equitable Financing – Community-Rated Contributions
Benchmark 5:	Equitable Financing – By Ability to Pay
Benchmark 6:	Value for Money – Clinical Efficacy
Benchmark 7:	Value for Money – Financial Efficiency
Benchmark 8:	Public Accountability
Benchmark 9:	Comparability
Benchmark 10:	Degree of Consumer Choice

*Adapted from Daniels *et al. Benchmarks of Fairness for Health Care Reform*, 1996.

Some of the benchmarks described by Daniels *et al.* are less central to debates in the UK than in the USA, and in our analysis we draw mainly on the first five. These deal principally with questions of access and financing in health care. We also recognise the importance of consumer choice, the tenth benchmark. Rawls' 'difference principle' provides a guide to thinking about the balance between individual choice and social equity. If I buy some aspirin, it does not materially affect anyone else's well-being – there is plenty more on the shop's shelves. However, if I can access hospital care faster than someone else by paying for it, it may result in someone else not receiving it. (Economists will recognise questions of rationing and externalities lurking beneath the surface. One way of thinking about the 'difference principle', admittedly somewhat simplified, is as a strategy for dealing with negative externalities.) We think this approach offers us a more useful way of thinking about equity than other frameworks, such as utilitarianism, which has informed much thinking about health care in the past.

One option for this book would be to follow Daniels *et al.* and score the UK and other health care systems on a set of measures reflecting each benchmark. For example, on the benchmark for universal access, the UK scores well overall, although the picture is marred by problems with access to care for dentistry, ophthalmic and other services. The nursing element of long-term care has also been a problem, with calls for the Labour Government to commit to universal provision of a basic package of free nursing care wherever it is needed.[19] Turning to equitable financing, the UK again scores well because the UK retains a predominantly tax-financed health care system. In addition, private medical insurance actually increases the equity of UK health care financing because it tends to be purchased by people on higher incomes, thus bringing the UK closer to the equity principle of financial contribution being related to the ability to pay (*see* Chapter 2). However, the major downside of this arrangement is that private medical insurance confers the advantage of faster access to hospital treatment, so that access is related to ability to pay rather than clinical need.

Our main purpose here, though, is different to that of Daniels *et al.* Whereas they were concerned with the equity of a whole health care system, we are concerned with the effects of the private sector within the UK system. There are simply too many holes in the data available about the equity effects of different parts of the UK health care system to allow us to mount a similar exercise, interesting though the results would be. Instead, we use the benchmarks heuristically, supported by quantitative data where it is available, to provide evidence about the equity of current arrangements.

We can also draw on experiences in other countries to highlight important aspects of the UK system. In other countries, policy-makers have devoted considerable effort to ensuring that, in overtly mixed public–private systems, the ability to pay does not confer undue advantages to the better-off, through faster access or better-quality treatment (*see* Chapter 6). There has been little equivalent effort in the UK, though the direction of government policy towards greater integration of public and private health care suggests that such effort needs to be made, and sooner rather than later.

In drawing on Rawls' arguments, we are aware that they are the subject of a very extensive critique. In the context of this book, the most important criticism is that his ideas are too abstract for application to real-world problems.[20] This is clearly true for some of the great questions of social justice. His ideas do not lead to practical policies for allocating benefits or other resources across a society. This criticism notwithstanding, we believe that the 'difference principle', combined with a transparent means of operationalising equity criteria, offers a clearer framework for thinking about equity in health care than any of the available alternatives.

Wider equity considerations

We are also aware that it would be possible to focus on other aspects of equity: for example, the equity of health outcomes or health status. Even though we will focus mainly on questions that relate to access and financing, it is important to note that developments in health care provision are set against a background of marked inequalities in illness and income in the UK. The Acheson report[21] set out the increase in inequalities in the incidences of major illnesses, such as coronary heart disease, between the richest and poorest in society during the past 25 years (*see* Figure 1.1).

If health care financing and provision develop in a way that tends to deny access to people on lower incomes (or other traditionally disadvantaged groups of people), then it can only increase the divisions between the 'haves' and 'have nots' in society. The Labour Government has made serious efforts in some areas of policy, such as the design of certain benefits, to reduce income inequalities. It would be a very great pity if these efforts were undermined by a failure to think through the consequences of health policies.

It is laudable to focus on long-term social goals, but the risk is that policy-makers may overlook positive changes they can make in the short term. We think that the current policy debate about private health care should focus on problems of access, for which more data are available, and whose effects are more immediate and more open to remedy. For example, the Government has estimated that some 2 million people who want NHS dental treatment are not able to access it. There is no doubt that some of this number will instead use private dental treatment and can afford to do so, but others will not be able to afford it. People with exemptions from payment for NHS dental treatment, who are typically on lower incomes and cannot afford to pay, are in effect being denied treatment. Surely, this is a problem that could be addressed by a government genuinely committed to universal access for basic primary care services.

Consumer protection

This principle seems straightforward, at least in comparison with equity, but there is more to it than meets the eye. For example, the National Consumer Council views its role as:

Figure 1.1 Standardised mortality rates, by Townsend quintile, males and females, England, 1993–95

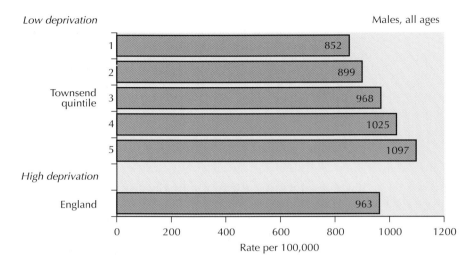

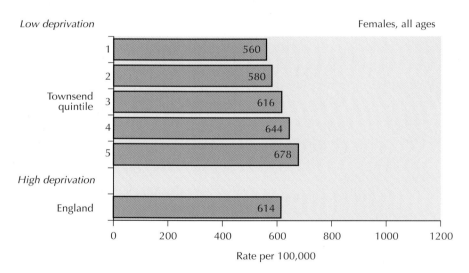

Source: Acheson D. *Independent Inquiry into Inequalities in Health,* 1999.

representing the interests of the consumers of goods and services of all kinds, whether publicly or privately supplied. We ensure that those who take decisions affecting consumers – and particularly policy-makers in Government, Parliament, industry, business and the professions – have a balanced and authoritative view of their users' interests before them.[22]

Ensuring that powerful institutions know their users' interests, however, could be thought paternalistic. It leaves users as powerless recipients of goods and services. Of course, consumers do need protection from dangerous and deceptive practices, but the first thought should be to inform consumers and enable them to exercise choice. Thus, consumer protection begins with policies that require providers, insurers and other agents to gather and make public information about their services and products, including cost and quality. This applies to both publicly and privately provided services. An example from California illustrates what is possible (*see* Table 1.2). There are public reports of patient ratings of clinical services, presented so that people can see which health plans offer the best services on a number of different dimensions, and whether or not ratings have improved or deteriorated since last year.

However, even if this type of public information were introduced in the UK, there would still be a need for the back-up provision of the more traditional forms of consumer protection. One cluster of protections involves inspections for safety, equipment performance and staffing, the subject of inspections in many industries. Another cluster of protections involves transparent systems for responding to complaints. It is important to examine these protections because there is evidence of unsafe and poor-quality care in private settings. The Health Committee of the House of Commons usefully gathered together a large volume of individual testimonies in its report on the regulation of private health care in 1999.[23] The report identified problems in a number of settings, including acute psychiatry, small specialist clinics such as those offering cosmetic surgery, and walk-in centres. The problems varied in their seriousness, but the Committee felt that the overall weight of evidence pointed strongly to the need to strengthen the most basic protections of consumer interests regarding the quality of care on offer.

Finally, we recognise that consumer protection issues are just as relevant to the NHS as to the private sector. Indeed, some of the most appalling treatment has been provided by the same individual working in both public and private sectors, as happened in the case of gynaecologist Rodney Ledward.[24] There are undoubtedly serious weaknesses in the quality of care provided in some parts of the NHS, and in the last few years both the Government and the professions have made proposals for improvement.[25] There are also problems with the NHS complaints mechanisms, which have received serious criticism.[26] If this book focuses on consumer issues in private health care, it is not because we think the NHS has got it right – far from it.

Table 1.2 Published patient satisfaction with health plans in California*

California health plans	Overall satisfaction		Interaction with physician				Access to care		Referral process			Member services	
	Satisfaction with health plan	Quality of care & services	Recommend to friend or family	Attention to what you say	Time with doctors & staff	Explanation of tests and procedures	Ease of choosing physician	Time b/w scheduling and visit	Authorisations have not delayed care	No difficulty receiving needed care	Ease of receiving referrals	No recent complaints	Staff able to answer questions
Aetna North	77	85▲	81	85▲	76▲	77▲	76▲	69▲	69	70▼	59	82	79
Aetna San Diego	81▲	83	84▲	81	74	76	76	70▲	71	81▲	58	86	88▲
Aetna South	76	77	77	74▼	66▼	71	67▼	60▼	61▼	71▼	52▼	83	84
Blue Cross/CaliforniaCare	78	80	80	79	70	75	70	59▼	66▼	77	57	85	79
Blue Shield	72▼	79	73▼	80	72	70	68▼	67	62▼	70▼	52	74▼	74▼
CareAmerica	73▼	73▼	76▼	72▼	64▼	68▼	66▼	60▼	64▼	73▼	51▼	84	87▲
CIGNA HealthCare Northern	78	83	83	84▲	75	73	71	69▲	74	78	62▲	79▼	79
CIGNA HealthCare San Diego	77	85▲	82	86▲	79▲	74	80▲	70▲	71	75	56	80▼	86▲
CIGNA HealthCare Southern	67▼	70▼	65▼	73▼	61▼	65▼	62▼	57▼	63▼	68▼	46▼	77▼	75▼
FHP/TakeCare	81▲	81	79	79	70	73	72	57▼	74	78	58	88▲	73▼
Foundation Health	69▼	79	70▼	80	74	72	66▼	71▲	61▼	69▼	56	80▼	67▼
Health Net	75	77▼	80	78	70	72	69	60▼	68	75	54	86	80
Health Plan of the Redwoods	79	90▲	83▲	89▲	84▲	81▲	87▲	79▲	76▲	80▲	60▲	87▲	89▲
Kaiser Permanente Northern	85▲	81	87▲	80	68▼	74	69	57▼	90▲	87▲	60	92▲	83
Kaiser Permanente Southern	84▲	80	90▲	79	71	75	72	58▼	88▲	87▲	62▲	92▲	89▲
Lifeguard	84▲	88▲	88▲	88▲	80▲	79▲	81▲	77▲	75▲	78	62▲	85	86▲
Maxicare	79	76▼	80	78	68▼	71	70	57▼	70	78	56	87▲	79
National Health Plan	★	★	★	★	★	★	★	★	★	★	★	★	★
Omni Healthcare	74▼	81	78	82	75	74	75	68	69	77	58	81	82
PacifiCare	80	78	85▲	77▼	67▼	72	71	55▼	71	78	56	87▲	86▲
Prudential HealthCare HMO	74	76▼	76▼	76▼	70▼	69	69	64	66▼	78	58	84	79
United HealthCare	☆	☆	☆	☆	☆	☆	☆	☆	☆	☆	☆	☆	☆
Average of all plans surveyed	77	80	80	80	72	73	72	65	71	77	57	84	81

00▲ = above average   **00** = average   **00▼** = below average

☆ = Response rate for this plan did not meet minimum reporting threshold (25 per cent)

★ = Plan did not participate in National Committee for Quality Assurance (NCQA) Member Survey

*Source: Light D W. *Effective Commissioning: lessons from purchasing in American managed care*, 1998.

Origins of the public–private divide

In the development of UK health care during the 20th century, the creation of the NHS represented a fundamental change in funding and provision.[27,28] Services that were once paid for from a mix of limited social insurance, charitable donations, savings schemes and out-of-pocket payment were made free to everyone. A system that was fragmented and inequitable was replaced with one that was better integrated and more equitable, at least in terms of financing. The break with the past was, however, far from complete. The structures created at the foundation of the NHS embodied compromises with powerful interests, and much of the activity outside the NHS today has its origins in the pre-NHS world.

Following the Royal Commission on the Poor Laws and Relief of Distress in 1909, and the introduction of National Health Insurance after 1911, the State began to guarantee the provision of basic services, particularly to poorer people. This process was developed and extended to new groups of people until the 1940s, when some 25 million people – or about a half of the population – were covered to some degree.[29] At this point, National Health Insurance covered general practitioner care, but not hospital-based or other institutional care. Working people were covered, but not their dependants – including most women and children – with the coverage varying according to the kind of work people did.

One result of National Health Insurance was a decline in the friendly societies and other payment schemes that had developed during the 19th and early part of the 20th centuries. They retained a role, however, because the exclusions to National Health Insurance were so extensive, and became a crucial source of income for the voluntary hospitals. It was estimated that, in the 1930s, half of all people covered by National Health Insurance also had savings plans for themselves and their dependants.[30] The importance of friendly societies declined substantially with the introduction of free NHS primary and secondary care services, though they did not disappear. The modern successors of those friendly societies still exist, in the form of mutual organisations that offer health cash plans. These plans have become increasingly popular in recent years, and are currently held by around 6 million people (*see* Chapter 3).

Private medical insurance, specifically for the costs of health care, was also available before 1948. BUPA and PPP Healthcare, now the largest and second largest private medical insurance organisations respectively, trace their origins back to the 1940s. They were set up to cater for people on higher incomes who wanted to offset the increasing costs of health care. They developed in parallel with the friendly societies and other associations that offered low-cost cash products. At the founding of the NHS, they were reduced to a fringe role. The market for non-NHS care – which typically meant hospital-based care – grew only slowly until the 1970s. Both health cash plans and private medical insurance highlight the point that co-existence of state and private financing of health care has a long history.

Provision of hospital care in the years before the creation of the NHS in 1948 was a patchwork of public, private and voluntary provision. There was a network of some 2000 municipal hospitals, and about 1000 voluntary hospitals, both types varying in size from small cottage hospitals upwards. Funding was a problem, particularly for the voluntary hospitals, throughout the early part of the 20th century. One consequence of these financial crises was renewed charitable activity, resulting in additional revenue to existing voluntary hospitals, as well as the development of new private hospitals with charitable status. This led to the establishment of groups, such as the Nuffield Hospitals, which today is the third largest private hospital provider and retains charitable status. It was also partly due to the perilous financial state of many voluntary hospitals, which opened the door to the NHS in 1948.

With the growing importance of public financing of health services, the relationship between the State and the medical profession became increasingly important for the development of both finance and provision. For our account, the most interesting aspects of the relationship concern the profession's desire to maintain its independence throughout the 20th century, manifested by the insistence of GPs on becoming independent contractors to the State rather than salaried employees, and its resistance to direction from lay people (e.g. sitting on NHS panels) concerning the type of work carried out by doctors. There was also an increasing separation between general practitioner and hospital services, such that the trajectories of the two led to different outcomes at the founding of the NHS.[31]

By the late 1930s, hospital consultants and specialists typically held 'honorary' part-time posts, but also maintained private practices. GPs treated employed people (mainly men) under the National Health Insurance scheme, but also maintained private practices, with non-insured people (mainly women and children) paying directly for treatment or via the friendly societies. This period also witnessed the creation of other services by the State, such as the district medical service which provided basic health services through local government to people outside the National Health Insurance scheme. Overall, a patchwork of state-funded and private medical practice was established, although it took different forms for different types of doctors.

The NHS: a new set of public–private relations

When the NHS was created, it did not represent a clean break with the past. Key elements of the health system were nationalised, including the great majority of hospitals. Elsewhere, however, there were adaptations of what had existed before, brokered by Aneurin Bevan and conditioned by a need to reassure and encourage a number of conservative, professional-interest groups into taking part in the new service. There was no single, blanket solution. There were, for example, different settlements arrived at with general practitioners and hospital doctors.[32] On the one hand, GPs were allowed to maintain their independent contractor status, though now on contract to a universal, tax-funded system. They effectively gave up private work, since their new contract with the NHS forbade them to offer their enrolled public patients any of the general medical services covered by the NHS in a private capacity. On the other hand, hospital consultants and specialists were given salaries but allowed to maintain parallel private practices. Private financing and provision of health care were consigned to a residual role serving a minority of the population, but they did not disappear. Table 1.3 lists some of the key public–private relationships created in the formative years of the NHS.

Table 1.3 Some long-standing public–private relationships

- General practitioners are independent contractors, not salaried employees
- Specialist doctors and other professionals can maintain NHS and private practices
- NHS pay beds, where hospitals retain a proportion of income and consultants charge separately for services
- Prescription and other user charges for NHS services (from 1951)
- Access to private treatment on the basis of ability to pay rather than need
- Reliance of the NHS on pharmaceutical and other industries to develop new products

Looking back over 50 years of the NHS, it is possible to see that some of the large-scale features of the compromise have remained remarkably stable.[33] Important details have changed over the years, but much of what was in place in 1946 is still there, and has important implications for policy-making today. This extends to relationships with private companies: from the start, the NHS depended on them to supply pharmaceuticals, medical equipment, and other products and services. It is a truism, therefore, to say that public–private relationships were built into the fabric of health care from the start of the NHS.

The creation of the NHS is not, however, the end of the story. There have been important changes in the boundaries of the NHS since 1948, which have come about in different ways. Prescription and dental charges were introduced in 1951 in an attempt to contain the growing NHS budget. A fee for NHS eye tests was introduced in 1989 by a Conservative Government, although this was subsequently removed in April 2000 for people aged 60 years and over by the Labour Government. The increase in private nursing home provision in the early 1980s appears to have been the unintentional consequence of changes in social security and other rules, but it has been accompanied by a major reduction in the provision of long-stay NHS hospital care for the very old, which has not been restored. At the same time, the NHS has continued to provide new treatments as they have become available and has greatly expanded the range of clinical services on offer. Thus, the NHS now offers a range of transplant services, minimally invasive therapies, and access to new classes of pharmaceuticals.

Two examples illustrate the ways in which NHS boundaries have changed over time. The first was the attempt to abolish NHS pay beds and rein in the private hospital sector in the 1970s. The Labour Government of the time was opposed to the existence of pay beds in NHS hospitals. Many MPs were ideologically opposed to privately funded care in general, even though it was small by today's standards, accounting for only 3 per cent of total health care expenditure, compared with approximately 16 per cent today. Barbara Castle, Secretary of State at the time, partly reflecting her links with NHS trade unions, made much of her desire to phase out pay beds. She famously entered into a confrontation with the political side of the medical profession. This period tends to be remembered now as the one in which Barbara Castle failed to remove NHS pay beds and was beaten back by the medical profession. However, the true sequence of events was more complicated. Mrs Castle was at loggerheads with the medical profession when Harold Wilson resigned as Prime Minister. He was succeeded by James Callaghan, who appointed David Ennals as Secretary of State for Health. He steered the Health Services Act of 1976 through Parliament, which sought to reduce and eventually remove NHS pay beds, and also to regulate the expansion of the private sector.[34]

The Health Services Board – in effect an early health service regulator – was set up to undertake the necessary tasks.

Attempts to reduce the numbers of pay beds were partially successful, with numbers falling from over 4000 in 1976 to 2800 by mid-1979. But this appears to have been the trigger for an increase in the size of the independent acute hospital sector, a classic case of an unintended consequence of policy-making. As Webster noted:

> If anything the policy of phasing out pay beds operated to stimulate growth in the private sector, and the Health Services Board found itself presiding over this expansion. Labour therefore failed in its objective to eliminate pay-beds from the NHS, and it succeeded in stimulating rather [than] repressing the private sector of health care.[35]

The episode reduced the role of the NHS in providing private beds, while showing that there was still an underlying demand for private health care. The latter was then provided for outside the NHS, since the Labour Government was reluctant to restrict freedom of choice outside the NHS. The Labour Government had sought to regulate the private sector, albeit in an incomplete manner, by focusing on provision of private care in the NHS, rather than regulating all health care provision and so ignoring the issue of finance. Nonetheless, for a brief period, Barbara Castle and David Ennals had acted as if they had some responsibility for all health care, and not just the NHS. However, their aim was ideological, attempting to 'purify' the NHS of any favouritism based on wealth rather than regulate the health care system as a whole.

When the Conservatives won the 1979 election, they disbanded the Health Services Board, but invested its powers in the Secretary of State.[36] These powers are still on the Statute Book, so that the Secretary of State has the powers to control the supply of health care, both in the NHS and outside it. Under Conservative administrations of the 1980s and 1990s, these powers were rarely exercised, while successive administrations have placed few restrictions in the path of private sector finance and provision.

The second example of shifting public–private boundaries concerns a major policy initiative – the NHS Review of 1989 – which led to the separation of purchasing and provision, the creation of NHS Trusts and GP fundholders, and a raft of other changes from 1991. (The development of the NHS internal market under successive Conservative Governments has been described in detail elsewhere.[37,38,39]) The creation of GP fundholders and health authorities with limited freedom to allocate resources outside the NHS was intended, at least in the early period of the reforms, to introduce competition between NHS and private providers as a mechanism to increase efficiency. In the view of some Conservatives, competition would in time lead to greater use of private health care and hence a mixed economy of provision. In the event, the volume of private health care purchased was small, the bulk of purchasing being from NHS providers.[40]

In the same period, income tax relief on private medical insurance premiums for people of 60 years of age and above was introduced, although the extent of relief was modest and the result was a correspondingly modest increase in the take-up of private medical insurance policies. Thus, most of the subsidy went to existing policyholders and was removed by the incoming Labour administration after 1997. Within the first two years of the start of the 'internal market' in 1991, the Government had judged that rapid introduction of an explicitly mixed economy of provision of health care was too risky politically. The Conservative regime was accused of wanting to dismantle the NHS, and in response slowed down the pace of change in order to regain voter confidence. This view, supported by some statements at the time, underlines the fact that successive Conservative Secretaries of State for Health believed in the principles underlying the NHS even if some of their colleagues may have been more lukewarm.[41]

During the same period in the 1990s, the private acute health sector grew, though not as fast as it had in the 1980s following the reduction in the number of NHS pay beds. The growth of private acute medicine after 1979 was in tune with Conservative thinking of the time. New private hospitals and clinics were opened as the Government relaxed some of the restrictions on building private facilities. Yet, at the same time, ministers seem to have been reluctant to champion private medicine directly. Representatives of private medical insurers and hospital providers have told us that Conservative ministers had been reluctant to engage with them, particularly during the period following the publication of the White Paper, *Working for Patients*, in 1989. The Conservatives seem to have had a love–hate relationship with both the NHS and private health care, and could not decide on the values that they felt should inform the design of a health care system. The electoral popularity of the NHS may also have influenced their actions, since even users of private health services generally support the existence of the NHS.[42]

Towards a mixed economy of provision

We are currently in the midst of another important phase in the development of public–private relations in the UK health system. The policy on private health care, both under the Conservatives and under Labour until 1999, was that there was no policy. Under Labour Secretary of State Frank Dobson (1997–99), the private sector was tolerated, but he preferred not to have to deal with it.[43] He argued that the NHS should become so good that no one should need to use privately funded care. However, after Alan Milburn had succeeded Frank Dobson in the summer of 1999, the ground was laid for the inclusion of the private sector in policy-making.[44]

There were five elements to the policy introduced by Milburn. First, there was a reinvigoration of the already strong political support for the NHS, backed by plans for unprecedented increases in real terms of NHS funding, as set out in the 2000 Budget. Second, the Government was prepared to concede that the NHS was far from perfect in practice and that 'seven deadly sins' built into the structure of the NHS since 1948 needed to be tackled through a thorough process of 'modernisation' (*see* Table 1.4).[45] Third, the NHS Plan of July 2000 confirmed that NHS funding could be used to purchase services from private providers. The NHS had used private hospitals for decades, but often in an *ad hoc* manner through local negotiation. According to the NHS Plan, the role of private providers would be formally recognised and private sector capacity would be considered in NHS planning decisions.[46] The nature of the NHS–private provider relationship was fleshed out a little in the Concordat published in Autumn 2000, which gave the green light to NHS Trusts to negotiate locally with private providers for intensive care, intermediate care and elective surgery.[47]

Table 1.4 The 'seven deadly sins' of the NHS*

- Capacity problems – 'the NHS has been under-funded for decades'
- An absence of national standards
- Difficulty of judging performance or a lack of information for clinicians and patients
- The absence of incentives to provide the best quality of care
- The absence of means to improve performance
- Rigid structural and professional demarcations
- Focus on treatment rather than prevention

*Adapted from Milburn A. *The New NHS – developing the NHS National Plan*. Speech. 18 May 2000.

Fourth, the Government stated clearly its analysis of the weaknesses of private medical insurance, arguing that it was both an inefficient and inequitable way of financing health care. Fifth, the Government signalled its intention to regulate the commitment of NHS consultants to both public and private clinical work in order to reduce the potentially conflicting incentives caused by the reliance of both public and private sectors on the same set of medical staff. The possible future direction of change is, therefore, towards publicly financed health care, but with a more mixed economy of provision.

The role of the King's Fund

At this point, it is proper to declare an interest. The King's Fund pre-dates the NHS, and provides another example of the persistence of the pre-1948 world in today's society. Established in 1897, the Fund has provided support for London hospitals in a variety of ways during the 20th century. Moreover, the Fund, together with the British Hospital Association, represented the interests of the voluntary hospitals in negotiation over the founding of the NHS. The Fund was at best wary of Aneurin Bevan's vision, preferring instead to support the continuing independence of voluntary hospitals, albeit with some public funding. As Prochaska noted:

> The Fund's officials read the White Paper [of 1944] with an eye to saving the hospitals from, in Lord Dawson's words, 'the stranglehold of local authorities'. It was also worried by the Government's cavalier use of the word 'free' in regard to future health provision … The Fund had assumed that the Treasury would only pay for the nation's health with the greatest reluctance. Thus for financial reasons alone, it believed voluntary traditions would continue to be vital.[48]

The King's Fund also played a role in the development of private medical insurance and health cash plans. Financial help was given in 1922 to set up HSA, now the largest health cash insurer, and in 1943 the Fund helped to establish the provident scheme Private Patients Plan (now PPP Healthcare). PPP was purchased by the general insurer, Guardian Royal Exchange, in 1997, thus giving up its mutual status, and Guardian Royal Exchange was in turn acquired by the French group, Axa, in 1999.

More recently, the Fund was home for some years to the Health Quality Service (HQS: formerly King's Fund Organisational Audit), part of whose business is accrediting private providers. Finally, to balance the account, the

Fund has for many years now provided the great majority of its resources to the NHS through grant-giving, development support and other activities. The Fund is now committed to the fundamental values of the NHS, namely to the equitable financing and provision of health care.

The structure of the book

Our starting point, in Chapter 2, is evidence about the different ways and means of financing and providing health care in the UK. It is possible to 'map' resource use and activity in different parts of the health care sector, and to investigate the nature of markets for different goods and services. The mapping exercise highlights the nature and extent of activity in private hospitals, and patterns of expenditure on other goods and services such as dentistry and complementary therapies. The mapping draws on published sources, particularly for quantitative evidence of the nature and scale of work in different sectors, and on interviews undertaken with representatives of private medical insurers, private providers of goods and services, regulators, and other relevant parties such as civil servants.

Chapter 3 continues the mapping of resource use and activity, but from the point of view of the individual. UK policy debates tend to omit consideration of products and services funded directly by individuals, especially outside the NHS. As we will see, this type of expenditure is far from negligible, though it can be difficult to quantify precisely. We then turn to other forms of payment for health care, such as health cash plans that are designed to enable people to pay for care out-of-pocket. We end by discussing the overall balance of individual and collective payments in the UK.

In Chapter 4, we investigate the boundaries between the public and private sectors. These boundaries are more numerous and more complicated than is generally realised. The fact that many hospital consultants work in both the NHS and private sectors is only part of the story. Many dentists undertake NHS and private work on the same premises. The NHS depends on privately owned and run pharmacies and opticians to deliver NHS services. Many of these public–private relationships would be difficult to change should any future government wish to do so, as they are long-standing and protected by powerful interests, including, but not limited to, the medical profession.

Another point of comparison is with overseas experiences, and these are discussed in Chapters 5 and 6. Several other countries belonging to the

Organisation for Economic Co-operation and Development (OECD) already make policies across the whole of their countries' health care systems, embracing public and private sectors. It is therefore valuable to look at their experiences, and we focus particularly on the USA, the Netherlands and Ireland, whose experiences, we believe, contain lessons for the UK. While systems in other countries are readily described as having 'mixed' arrangements for financing and provision – and see themselves in this way – the UK is typically deemed to be dominated by the NHS. As we show, the NHS remains the main provider of UK health care, but around 16 per cent of expenditure is now outside the NHS, and the UK is closer to some other European systems than is generally recognised.

In Chapter 7, we consider the regulation of health care. To a large extent, regulation reflects the fragmented approach to policy-making before 1999. Different regulators for the NHS and private health care systems execute their responsibilities in differing ways. Some of the regulators have considerable powers and are prepared to exercise them, but others have limited power and influence. The chapter comments on the extent to which current regulations protect or promote consumer interests. Finally, Chapter 8 draws together the themes and issues identified in earlier chapters, and looks at the possible implications for UK policy-making in the future. We consider the directions in which current policies seem to be taking us, and comment on the degree to which policies are, or could be, informed by equity considerations.

References

1   MacAskill E, Bowcott O. Furious NHS protester blocks Blair's path. *The Guardian* 2001; 17 May: 1.
2   Edghill S. Safe in their hands? *Good Housekeeping* 2000; July: 116–20.
3   Botched private surgery patients take NHS beds. *The Sunday Times* 1999; 11 April: 7.
4   Identical twins requiring identical heart surgery. *The Express* 1998; 29 December: 9.
5   HM Treasury. *Prudent for a Purpose: working for a stronger and fairer Britain*. HC 346. London: Stationery Office, 2000.
6   Timmins N. Blair in policy shift on private hospitals. *Financial Times* 2000; 29 February: 2.
7   Blair T. *Hansard* 2000; 22 March: col. 981.
8   Milburn A. *Reinventing Health Care. A Modern NHS versus a Private Alternative.* Speech at the London School of Economics. London, 20 December 1999.
9   Timmins N. NHS looks to private sector. *Financial Times* 2000; 15 June: 3.
10 Hood C. A management for all seasons? *Pub Admin* 1991; 69: 3–19.
11 Secretary of State for Health. *The NHS Plan: a plan for investment; a plan for reform.* Cm 4818-I. London: Stationery Office, 2000.

12 World Health Organisation. *World Health Report 2000*. Geneva: WHO, 2000: 36.

13 Light D. The practice and ethics of risk-rated health insurance. *JAMA* 1992; 267: 2503–8.

14 Williams B. Utilisation of National Health Service hospitals in England by private patients 1989–95. *Health Trends* 1997; 29: 21–5.

15 Acheson D. *Independent Inquiry into Inequalities in Health*. London: Stationery Office, 1999.

16 Rice T. *The Economics of Health Reconsidered*. Chicago: Health Administration Press, 1998.

17 Rawls J. *A Theory of Justice*. Princeton: Princeton University Press, 1971.

18 Daniels N, Light D, Caplan R. *Benchmarks of Fairness for Health Care Reform*. New York: Oxford University Press, 1996.

19 Secretary of State. *The Government's Response to the Royal Commission on Long-Term Care*. London: Stationery Office, 2000.

20 Kymlicka W. *Political Philosophy: a critical introduction*. New York: Oxford University Press, 1990.

21 Acheson D. *Independent Inquiry into Inequalities in Health*. London: Stationery Office, 1999.

22 National Consumer Council. *Self-regulation of Professionals in Health Care*. London: NCC, 1999.

23 Health Committee. *The Regulation of Private Medicine and Other Independent Healthcare*. 281-I. Session 1998–99. London: Stationery Office, 1999.

24 Ritchie J. *An Inquiry into Quality and Practice within the National Health Service arising from the Actions of Rodney Ledward*. London: Department of Health, 2000.

25 Donaldson L. *Supporting Doctors, Protecting Patients*. London: Department of Health, 1999.

26 Wallace H, Mulcahy L. *Cause for Complaint? An evaluation of the effectiveness of the NHS complaints procedure*. London: Public Law Project (Birkbeck College, University of London), 1999.

27 Webster C. *The Health Services Since the War*. Vol I. London: HMSO, 1988.

28 Rivett G. *From Cradle to Grave*. London: King's Fund, 1998.

29 Pater J. *The Making of the National Health Service*. Ch. 1. London: King Edward's Hospital Fund for London, 1981: 1–23.

30 Webster C. *The Health Services Since the War*. Vol I. Ch. 1. London: HMSO, 1988: 1–5.

31 Honigsbaum F. *The Division in British Medicine*. Ch. 30. London: Kogan Page, 1979: 340–56.

32 Ibid.

33 Mays N, Keen J. Will the fudge on equity sustain the NHS into the next millennium? *BMJ* 1998; 317: 66–9.

34 Webster C. *The Health Services Since the War*. Vol I. London: HMSO, 1988: 1.

35 Ibid.: 627.

36 *Health Services Act 1980*. London: HMSO, 1980.

37 Butler J. *Patients, Policies and Politics: before and after working for patients*. Buckingham: Open University Press, 1992.

38 Le Grand J, Mays N, Mulligan J-A, editors. *Learning from the NHS Internal Market – a review of the evidence*. London: King's Fund, 1998.

39 Light D. From managed competition to managed cooperation: theory and lessons from the British experience. *Milbank Quarterly* 1997; 75: 297–341.

40 Audit Commission. *What the Doctor Ordered: a study of GP fundholders in England and Wales*. London: HMSO, 1996.

41 Ham C. *The Politics of NHS Reform 1988–97: metaphor or reality?* London: King's Fund, 2000.

42 Calnan M, Cant M, Gabe M. *Going Private*. Buckingham: Open University Press, 1993.

43 Health Committee. *The Regulation of Private Medicine and Other Independent Healthcare*. 281-I. Session 1998–99. London: Stationery Office, 1999.

44 Milburn A. *Reinventing Health Care. A Modern NHS versus a Private Alternative*. Speech at the London School of Economics. London, 20 December 1999.

45 Milburn A. *The New NHS – developing the NHS National Plan*. Speech at the Royal College of Surgeons. London, 18 May 2000.

46 Secretary of State for Health. *The NHS Plan: a plan for investment, a plan for reform*. Cm 4818-I. London: Stationery Office, 2000.

47 Department of Health. *For the Benefit of Patients – a concordat with the private and voluntary health care provider sector*. London: Department of Health, 2000.

48 Prochaska F. *Philanthropy and the Hospitals of London: The King's Fund 1897–1990*. Ch. 6. Oxford: Clarendon Press, 1992: 82–90.

Chapter 2

Public and private funding in the UK

Introduction

At least until the current furore over public–private partnerships, most discussion of health policy in the UK assumed that the NHS is the only health care provider. This is far from being the case, and there is a substantial, diverse health care system outside the NHS. The NHS and health care markets outside it have grown up separately over the last 50 years, and there have been few attempts to co-ordinate either financing, provision or regulation between the two. This chapter describes the contours of private health care, and shows how private health care markets are related to patterns of provision within the NHS despite their separate development.

The chapter starts with a brief outline of events before and after the founding of the NHS in 1948 to show how key institutions, relationships and boundaries evolved. Then, two distinct ways of viewing public–private relations are presented, to identify resource flows and patterns of resource use. Since our main interest in this chapter is in private financing and provision, most of the discussion focuses on arrangements outside the NHS. However, relevant NHS statistics are presented to provide a context and basis for comparison with private sector activities and costs.

Two views of public–private relations

To help shape the descriptive material in Chapters 2 and 3, it is helpful to view the relationships between public and private health care in two contrasting ways. The first view focuses on the nature of funding, and distinguishes between public and private financing of services, in addition to public and private provision.[1,2] Table 2.1 captures this distinction and gives illustrative examples of each combination.

The second view is based on the distinction between individual and collective payment for services. Some health services are paid for from common or shared funds, including general taxation, National Insurance and private medical insurance (i.e. some form of risk-pooling), while other services are paid for

Table 2.1 Public and private financing and provision of health care

	Public financing	Private financing
Public provision	NHS services	NHS pay beds, NHS user charges
Private provision	NHS Concordats for elective surgery and elements of intermediate care, some mental health services	Privately provided services financed through out-of-pocket payment, loans or private medical insurance. Contributory schemes used for private dental and other services

directly by individuals out of their own pockets, including from their savings (i.e. no risk-pooling). With the persistence of user charges for NHS services and the rise of out-of-pocket payment for private health care, individual payments for health care merit particular attention and are dealt with at length in Chapter 3. There are other dimensions of the public–private divide that have practical and ideological implications, such as who *owns* the facilities in which care is provided and who *controls* what goes on and how this control is exercised. Much less important, in practice, is the distinction between for-profit and not-for-profit providers.

The rest of this chapter is devoted to examining the first view – public versus private financing and provision. It examines each of the four quadrants in Table 2.1 in turn, starting with the publicly financed and provided quadrant. While it is not our purpose here to provide a detailed assessment of the current performance of the NHS, we will highlight key data about costs and activity, in order to sketch out the 'public' side of the public–private divide, and to provide a basis for comparison with the scale of private costs and activity.

The balance between public and private finance

First, what is the overall balance of public and private financing? Propper notes that there are four main sources of health care financing in the UK (as in most OECD countries), namely, general taxation, social insurance (i.e. National Insurance contributions), private medical insurance and direct payment out-of-pocket. OECD figures show that general taxation and National Insurance accounted for 84 per cent of expenditure in 1997, with 16 per cent financed through private medical insurance and out-of-pocket payments.[3]

It is interesting to note that the percentage of total UK health care expenditure financed and provided by the NHS has declined slowly over the last 30 years. Leaving aside the changes in the pattern of services delivered (*see* Chapter 4), the decline has been from about 97 per cent of public finance for health care in the 1960s to around 84 per cent at present. The UK still has a predominantly tax-financed system, however, and Figure 2.1 gives the sources of finance for the NHS in England for 1998–99. Around 90 per cent of gross NHS spending in England was met from two sources, namely the Consolidated Fund – general taxation – and the NHS element of National Insurance contributions.

Figure 2.1 NHS sources of financing, 1998–99 (Total £42,131m)*

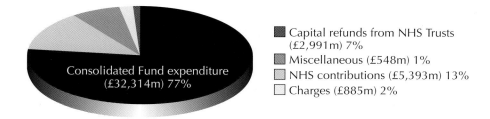

Consolidated Fund expenditure (£32,314m) 77%

■ Capital refunds from NHS Trusts (£2,991m) 7%
■ Miscellaneous (£548m) 1%
□ NHS contributions (£5,393m) 13%
□ Charges (£885m) 2%

*Source: Department of Health. *Departmental Report 2000,* 2000.

The balance between public and private financing and provision is not the same for all services, and it is useful to identify differences between services in the balance of public–private funding so that the boundaries between the two can be seen more clearly. Unfortunately, this is not a straightforward exercise because there are important gaps in our information about both NHS and private activity and costs. Because of these gaps, it is necessary to express the public–private balance in different units for different services. Table 2.2 provides a number of illustrative examples of the mix (using the four quadrants from Table 2.1). It is interesting to note that the NHS is by far the dominant provider of some services, such as accident and emergency and maternity services, but the minority provider of services such as continuing nursing care. The extent of private provision of dental treatments and some types of elective surgery is also greater than is generally recognised. General medical and general dental services are not straightforward to categorise according to the scheme in Table 2.1; although legally the providers are 'private', they operate in many ways as if they were part of the NHS. This is particularly true of GPs, who are regarded – and regard themselves – as a key pillar of the NHS.

Table 2.2 Patterns of financing: summary of selected services*

Service	Year	Basis of partition	Public finance		Private finance	
			public provision (%)	private provision (%)	public provision (%)	private provision (%)
Elective surgery carried out on UK residents	1997	Cases	86.4	0.2	1.5	11.9
Abortions performed in England on UK residents (a)	1997	Cases	50	22	Small	28
Maternity care of UK residents	1995	Births	99	Small	Small	1
Long-term care of elderly people in residential or nursing home settings	1998	Cash	26	35	2	37
Acute psychiatric treatment	1998	Beds	91	3	Small	6
Psychiatric rehabilitation and long-term nursing or residential home care of mentally ill people	1997	Beds	33	67	Small	Small
General practice	1996	Consultations	97	0	0	3
General dental services in England (c)	1996–97	Cash	56.8	0	23.2	20.0
General ophthalmic services (b)	1998	Eyesight tests	53	0	0	47
Pharmaceuticals	1995	Cash	61	0	5	35

*Adapted from Laing and Buisson. *Laing's Healthcare Market Review 1999–2000*, 1999. Amended with data from other sources.
(a) Office for National Statistics. *Abortion Statistics 1997.* Table 21 (Figures for England only), 1998: 27.
(b) Federation of Ophthalmic and Dispensing Opticians. *Optics at a Glance*, 1999.
(c) Department of Health (personal communication).

Public financing and provision

The top left quadrant in Table 2.1 covers services that are both financed and provided publicly. It is still the norm for people to go into an NHS hospital when they need to, or to be visited by a community nurse, with the care provided free at the point of delivery by public sector-employed staff. The NHS is available to the whole population of the UK. However, it is worth noting that it is far more common for NHS users to visit their general practice, which is funded but not owned by the NHS. Table 2.3 presents high level data about NHS spending and activity in England. Table 2.4 shows the Government's expenditure plans contained in the Government's 2000 Budget, which projected average real increases of 6.1 per cent per annum in real terms in the NHS budget for England over the four years to 2004. The figures are subject to the usual caveats in Treasury forecasts, notably the rate of growth in the economy. Nevertheless, the figures signal the extent of the Government's material support for the NHS.

Table 2.3 NHS activity and expenditure in England

| | Annual turnover | |
	1997–98	1998–99
Ordinary and day-case admissions (1000s) (1)	4,771	N/A
Expenditure (turnover £ million) (2)		
Hospital, community health, family health (discretionary), and related services	30,025	31,933
Family health services	3,846	3,940
Other services	513	478
Total	**34,664**	**36,612**

(1) Health Committee. *Public Expenditure on Personal Health and Social Services 1999,* 1999: 121.
(2) Department of Health. *The Government's Expenditure Plans 2000–2001,* 2000: 84.

Table 2.4 NHS Spending in the UK, £ billion in current prices, financial year 2000–01*

	1998 –99	1999 –2000	2000 –01	2001 –02	2002 –03	2003 –04	Average
Expenditure	45.1	49.3	54.2	58.6	63.5	68.7	
Year-on-year real growth	–	–	7.4%	5.6%	5.6%	5.6%	7.1%

*Adapted from HM Treasury. *Prudent for a Purpose,* 2000.

Private financing and provision

The bottom right quadrant of Table 2.1 and the final column of Table 2.2 comprise services that are privately financed and provided. The single largest expenditure is on private acute health care (mostly elective surgery), which totals some £2.5 billion per annum. Treatment is paid for primarily through private medical insurance (70 per cent of the market) and individuals paying for treatment directly (20 per cent). The NHS also purchases services to a value of about 5 per cent of the total, with the remaining 5 per cent coming from a variety of sources, including patients from overseas.[4] Private medical insurance and self-payment are supplementary payments over and above tax and National Insurance contributions. They focus primarily on elective procedures, and typically do not cover emergency care, though emergency care may be covered if it is provided in either a private or NHS hospital on a private basis). Very little primary care is purchased privately in the UK.

It is useful to think of this part of the UK health care market for the most part in terms of three main actors, namely, insurers, hospitals (which employ many staff directly) and independent contractors who provide clinical services, the most important by far being hospital consultants.

Private financing: private medical insurance

The market for private medical insurance is dominated by a small number of companies, with the leading five companies taking around 88 per cent of the market:[5] the five are BUPA, PPP, WPA, Norwich Union and Prime. The remaining 12 per cent of the market is shared between about 20 companies. Until recently, the sector was dominated by mutual (non-profit) organisations, but PPP is now owned by the private for-profit general insurance firm Axa. The market is now split about half and half between mutuals and for-profit firms, with BUPA contributing to about 40 per cent of the mutual figure.

For most of its history, private medical insurance in the UK has been a simple product, at least in concept. Individuals or companies take out annual policies, which typically cover selected inpatient, day-case and outpatient treatments. If people fall ill, and the likely required treatment is covered by their policy, they are referred by their NHS GP to a private consultant for an initial consultation followed by private elective treatment at a private hospital by the same specialist. Hospitals and consultants will undertake their work and (separately) send their bills to the insurer, which will pay them as long the policy covers the work done. (Note that in the traditional arrangement, which is still common, any additional work undertaken by doctors that is not covered by the insurance results in a separate bill, which is sent to the patient.) Traditionally, both hospital and consultant have charged the insurer fees-for-service (though this is changing, as will be outlined later). The insurers' premiums to individuals and to companies reflect the costs of reimbursing the providers, internal administration and marketing costs, as well as profits for for-profit private firms or surpluses for business development for mutuals. The risks of the population of people with policies are pooled, and individuals make claims against this pool of cash. Private medical insurance has, therefore, historically been a form of indemnity insurance, where the insurer is a funder rather than an active purchaser of services.

How much is spent and who has private medical insurance?

Table 2.5 shows the sums spent on private medical insurance policies up to 1998. About half of all policies, by insurance policy income, are paid for by companies and the remainder by individuals. It can be cheaper to obtain cover through an employer than as an individual or family, especially if the insured works in a white-collar occupation with lower risk. Policies can be written for individuals and for families, and it is typical for a company employee to have private medical insurance as a fringe employment benefit and to have his or her family covered by the same policy.

Table 2.5 Trends in PMI subscription income and real growth by sector, 1989–99*

Year	Company-paid subscription income at current prices (£ million)	Real growth (%) in company-paid PMI subscription income (deflated by RPI)	'Other' subscription income at current prices (£ million)	Real growth (%) in 'other' PMI subscription income (deflated by RPI)
1989	498	–	453	–
1990	582	6.7	525	5.9
1991	671	8.9	608	9.4
1992	758	9.0	701	11.0
1993	777	0.8	763	7.2
1994	776	−2.4	829	6.1
1995	812	1.1	884	3.0
1996	882	6.1	963	6.4
1997	931	2.3	1038	4.5
1998	1008	4.7	1034	−3.6
1999	1075	5.1	1098	4.5

*Adapted from Laing and Buisson. *Laing's Healthcare Market Review 2000–2001*, 2000.

Eleven-and-a-half per cent of the population is covered by private medical insurance,[6] many of whom are employers, managers and professionals, other non-manual workers and self-employed people (*see* Table 2.6). It is relatively rare for people on lower incomes to have private medical insurance. People aged 45–64 years are most likely to be covered and people over 75 years least likely. The Office for National Statistics (ONS) reports that:

> *Around a sixth of non-retired couple households are covered by private health insurance and, on average, they spend £423 per year. Only one in ten retired couple households are members of private schemes but those who are spend an average of £779 per year.*[7]

Table 2.6 UK households covered by private health insurance by socio-economic group of head of household, 1996–97*

Socio-economic group	Percentage (%)
Professionals, employers and managers	17.2
Intermediate non-manual	15.1
Junior non-manual	7.7
Skilled manual	6.7
Semi-skilled and unskilled manual	4.8
Self-employed	13.6
Retired[1]	7.0
Unoccupied[2]	4.8
TOTAL	**11.5**

[1] Males aged 65 and over and females aged 60 and over who are not economically inactive.
[2] Males aged under 65 and females aged under 60 who are not working, nor actively seeking work.
* Adapted from Office for National Statistics. *Social Trends 29*, 1999.

The ONS figures include some non-private medical insurance spending, including spending on permanent health insurance and critical illness insurance. (These are products designed to provide income when people are ill or disabled, rather than pay for health care, and are not discussed here.) The ONS figures are therefore higher than for private medical insurance alone, but provide an indication of the levels of individual spending.

Table 2.7 shows the trend in the number of people covered by private medical insurance policies, distinguishing between insurance taken out by companies for employees and their dependants and 'other' policies, which are principally those taken out by individuals to cover themselves and their families, either

Table 2.7 Numbers of subscribers and people covered by private medical insurance (PMI)*

Year	Company-paid PMI		Other PMI (individual and employee)		Total PMI subscribers (millions)	Total persons covered by PMI (millions)	Proportion of population with PMI (%)
	Subscribers (million)	Persons covered	Subscribers (million)	Persons covered			
1989	1.833	3.927	1.207	2.282	3.040	6.209	10.8
1990	1.974	4.213	1.271	2.411	3.246	6.625	11.5
1991	1.911	4.057	1.321	2.497	3.233	6.554	11.3
1992	1.985	4.120	1.292	2.401	3.277	6.521	11.2
1993	2.018	3.853	1.263	2.309	3.282	6.162	10.6
1994	1.975	4.069	1.304	2.347	3.279	6.416	11.0
1995	1.964	4.024	1.342	2.392	3.306	6.416	10.9
1996	1.953	3.976	1.375	2.446	3.328	6.422	10.9
1997	2.039	4.186	1.327	2.271	3.366	6.457	10.9

*Adapted from Laing and Buisson. *Private Medical Insurance Market Sector Report,* 1999.

directly with an insurer or through entry to a voluntary scheme (which might be offered as an option by an employer). During the 1980s, there was a sustained increase in the size of the private acute insurance sector. After 1990, the situation became more complicated. Following contraction of the market during the severe recession of the early 1990s, growth was modest and did not seem to be helped by the modest income tax relief introduced in 1991. In 1997, the Labour Government removed the tax relief and introduced new general insurance taxes to take effect in 2000, but recent reports suggest that the number of policies purchased has increased over the last two years.

Insurance premiums have continued to increase in price faster than the rate of general inflation, and there is a widespread view within the industry that the market for private medical insurance is effectively saturated. The number of claims made has continued to increase (*see* Table 2.8), so that costs have eaten into income from premiums. Still, individual subscribers get back only 79 per cent of their premiums in benefits, while insurers keep 21 per cent for salaries, marketing, administration and profits. While this is 'better' than in 1995, when subscribers got back only 74 per cent of their premiums in benefits, subscribers did better in 1990 when they got back 84 per cent. Representatives of some insurers told us that many companies were losing money, although this was not obvious in company accounts. Equally, we were told that some firms remain profitable, but again, relevant figures were not available.

Table 2.8 Trends in private medical insurance (PMI) claims incurred and real growth (as indicated by deflation with retail price index (RPI)*

Year	Company-paid claims incurred at current prices (£ million)	Real growth (%) company-paid claims incurred (deflated by RPI)	'Other' PMI claims incurred at current prices (£ million)	Real growth (%) in 'other' PMI claims incurred (deflated by RPI)
1989	440	–	372	–
1990	540	12.2	440	8.0
1991	604	5.6	519	11.4
1992	642	2.5	553	2.8
1993	638	–2.2	578	2.8
1994	667	2.1	618	4.3
1995	711	3.0	658	3.0
1996	756	3.9	723	7.3
1997	793	1.7	768	2.8
1998	869	5.9	810	3.8
1999	928	5.2	866	5.3

*Adapted from Laing and Buisson. *Laing's Healthcare Market Review 2000–2001*, 2000.

Types of private medical insurance policies and extent of cover

UK private medical insurance insurers use two main ways of calculating policy premiums for individuals. Both are based on the premise that most people can be insured as long any pre-existing conditions are identified and excluded. In the UK, insurers are unwilling to insure people for their pre-existing conditions on the grounds that such conditions represent a known future cost and, therefore, a predictable 'loss' to the insurer. However, pre-existing conditions *are* covered by insurers in many other countries, with consequently treatment costs varying very widely between insured people. In these countries, where private medical insurance plays a bigger part in providing people's primary form of insurance against the costs of ill health, insurers are regulated in a variety of ways – which are unknown in the UK 'double-cover' private medical insurance market – to ensure that discrimination is minimum against people with chronic conditions so that they can obtain adequate cover. For example, many countries require private insurers to guarantee renewal of cover to individuals. In the UK, private insurers can always rely on the existence of the NHS to fulfil this function, thereby limiting their exposure to risk.

One technique by which insurers deal with pre-existing risks is 'moratorium' underwriting, where the individual's general health status is not formally assessed, but the individual is required to declare any pre-existing conditions before acceptance by the insurer. If the policyholder develops a need for care which the insurer can show to have existed before the policy was taken out and which was not declared though it could reasonably have been known to the patient, the care is not covered under the policy. In the case of declared conditions, the policyholder cannot generally claim for treatment of a pre-existing condition for as long as two years from the start of the policy, though he or she may be covered after this period.

The other type of policy is one where people are explicitly rated according to their risk profiles on the basis of a medical examination, so that the characteristics of individuals are included in the calculation of premiums. Individuals must declare pre-existing conditions, which, again, are excluded from policies.

In both cases, a scale of fees is calculated, which increase with age and rise steeply as one reaches and passes 65 years of age. Risk-rated policies are more difficult and costly for insurers to write since they involve screening individuals for risk rather than inferring risk from demographic data and other prognostic factors, but they have the advantage from the insurers' perspective of enabling discrimination between people with higher and lower health risks. From the patients' perspective, they are advantageous to healthier people, who may well be offered a lower quote compared to a moratorium policy. Equally, they are disadvantageous to less healthy people (assuming that the medical examination is revealing), who are most likely to claim and whose premiums are higher to reflect their greater health risks. Risk-related policies are more commonly sold than moratorium policies, but both types of policy are actively marketed by the industry. (The reservations of the Office of Fair Trading (OFT) concerning moratorium policies are discussed in Chapter 7.) This discussion of the basis of premiums setting emphasises that private medical insurance in the UK is designed to be selective rather than universal, and that selection is on the basis of both the ability to pay and the range of treatments covered.

Private medical insurers in the UK typically choose to cover those treatments and procedures that enable them to make a profit (or surplus, in the case of mutuals); private medical insurance does not therefore provide comprehensive coverage. People who have insurance have double cover because they insure for services on top of their payment of the tax and National Insurance contributions that finance the NHS. They are in effect paying for the privilege of faster access, more time and attention, and greater convenience for elective procedures, compared with their availability on the NHS. This contrasts with countries with social insurance-based systems such as the Netherlands (*see* Chapter 6), which do not permit insurers to compete selectively with the basic universal system.

Insurance was historically designed to cover hospital-based care, and it still mainly does so today. In most cases, insurance policies offer full coverage for acute elective inpatient treatment and for outpatient consultations if they lead to inpatient treatment. There are many important exclusions, however, including accident and emergency care and maternity care within the hospital sector – less than 1 per cent of hospital births are outside NHS hospitals[8] – almost all chronic and long-term treatments, and most GP and other community-based services. The exclusion of the great bulk of GP services means that, in practice, the most frequent encounters with health services are excluded.

The nature of NHS consultants' contracts means that there is a service available that can be paid for, and which offers advantages of speed and convenience. The nature of acute elective work is sufficiently predictable for insurance companies to know how often people in a population are likely to need treatment and the usual range of costs involved, while the costs of many treatments are high enough for people to need some way of 'smoothing out' payments.

By the same token, services which are not covered exhibit characteristics that make them a less attractive proposition for 'double-cover' insurers. Some services do not cost much and can easily be bought for cash (*see* Chapter 3 for more information). Others, such as pregnancy and childbirth, expose the insurer to a high risk of adverse selection (i.e. the patient has prior knowledge not available to the insurer of her intention of having a baby). The reasons for general practice being unavailable under private medical insurance are not so obvious, but include the presence of a free NHS service with short waits that is perceived to be at least good enough to make the private option unattractively expensive. In addition, the current national GP contract with the NHS means that GPs cannot offer general medical services (GMS) to their NHS-enrolled patients.

Selling private medical insurance

The great majority of private medical insurance sales to individuals involve people dealing directly with an insurer rather than through a broker. The sales may come about through direct advertising – including television advertising – and via direct sales forces employed by the insurers. Most companies now have web sites with details, though usually not prices, of their policies. Relatively few policies are sold through financial intermediaries, partly because the commission rates available make it a relatively unattractive product to sell.

The situation is different for policyholders who are covered by company policies. For these schemes, where large numbers of people are covered under one policy, the underwriting process is often waived and employees' pre-existing conditions disregarded since there is frequently sufficient commonality of risk among workers in similar jobs in the same industry for the insurer to be able to predict the claims profile in advance, with greater confidence than in the general public. In addition, people covered by company policies tend to be healthier than individual policyholders. For one thing, they will all be of working age and, for another, they will tend to be of below-average risk for their ages since they will include individuals who have few or no personal grounds for regarding themselves sufficiently at risk of ill health to have bothered to take out individual private medical insurance. In the market for company-paid insurance, about 75 per cent of policies are arranged through intermediaries. This intermediary market has grown in recent years, apparently in response to the presence of more insurers offering more types of policies, and perhaps also because of greater cost awareness on the part of company purchasers.

A representative of a large company which offers cover to several hundred of its senior employees told us that they had looked progressively more closely at the value of this perk over the last five years. Once, it was a perk that could be absorbed into company costs with relative ease. Companies saw clear advantages in fast access to treatment, as they could get employees back to work as soon as possible. However, high prices were now making private medical insurance more difficult to justify. Premiums for companies are typically in the range £300–£500 per employee per year, compared with £800–£1200 for an individual policy.

Cost pressures and limits to growth of the private medical insurance market

Part of the reason why the market for private medical insurance appears to have stalled is that insurers' costs have been increasing faster than the rate of general inflation as insurers have found it difficult to contain costs and premiums.[9] One reason for this has been that the private medical fees charged by consultants have been rising faster than general inflation in recent years; hence the attraction of self-insurance (out-of-pocket payment), which is discussed in the next chapter.

A second reason for cost increases is that the coverage of private medical insurance policies has widened in the last ten years, perhaps as a way of competing for a larger share of a largely static market, with a clear trend towards more complex procedures. These include coronary bypasses and knee joint replacements. The highest volumes undertaken are for less costly investigations, particularly endoscopies. The net effect of the increased range of coverage, together with escalating charges, has been to push up insurers' costs. In theory, insurers could continue to cover a restricted range of procedures and seek to keep costs down, but we were told that the market pressures were all the other way, towards increased coverage. Insurers have responded by segmenting the market by developing a spectrum of policies, ranging from low-cost or restricted-coverage policies at one end of the market to high-cost and broader-coverage policies at the other.

Table 2.9 Procedure costs, 1996*

Procedure	Hospital	Surgeon	Anaesthetist	Total
Hip replacement (including prosthesis)	6686	755	290	7751
Wisdom tooth extraction	644	310	135	1089
Hernia	1021	320	140	1481
D&C	664	155	130	949

*Adapted from Office of Fair Trading. *Health Insurance*, 1996.

Furthermore, although the number of subscribers is roughly static, the number of claims has been increasing (*see* Table 2.8), presumably in part because of the greater number of procedures that are now covered. The abolition of tax relief for people over 60 years of age in the 1997 Budget also increased premiums. Premiums are likely to be increased further by the increase in Insurance

Premium Tax from 4 per cent to 5 per cent, and the classification of private medical insurance (along with all other general insurance products) as a benefit in kind, and therefore incurring National Insurance contributions from the year 2000. BUPA experienced an average increase in premiums of 14 per cent for 2000, presumably reflecting these tax changes along with other cost pressures.

The result is that there are substantial cost pressures in the private medical insurance and associated private provider market. It is not surprising, then, to find insurers responding by adopting techniques from US managed care in an attempt to limit costs and premiums increases (*see* Chapter 4). For example, PPP Healthcare has developed preferred-provider networks, whereby patients may only go to a list of approved hospitals that have agreed to accept reduced payments from the insurer in return for inclusion on the list and thus the guarantee of a certain level of work and therefore income. BUPA has developed a scheme of 'clinical-care profiling', in which 'best-practice' profiles for all common treatments and their estimated costs have been developed. Profiling also enables the quality of care to be monitored. These developments may benefit patients, partly through closer monitoring of quality, and partly by leading to fixed, all-inclusive prices for treatments in approved hospitals, so that patients do not get a nasty surprise in the form of an extra bill from the consultant or the hospital after their stay. The latter signals a movement away from the traditional fee-per-item-of-service arrangements in the private sector. It seems likely to reduce inequities within the population of private patients.

Extension into niche markets at the limits of the NHS

A different response to cost pressures is for insurers to extend coverage into new markets. Whenever coverage has been extended, this seems partly to reflect judgements that attractive new services would not be covered comprehensively by the NHS (e.g. some complementary therapies) or that the NHS was withdrawing *de facto* from providing its previous level of service (e.g. dentistry).

Insurance companies have explored niche areas outside traditional hospital services in recent years as follows:

- The leading insurers offer limited cover for physiotherapy. The conditions for qualifying for treatment vary between policies. In some policies, the treatment must follow a hospital episode, while others require only a GP referral (the NHS attempts to offer access in both circumstances).

- Complementary therapies are covered by selected schemes. They tend to be included in the higher-cost personal schemes and excluded from lower-cost and company schemes.
- PPP, BUPA and other companies offer separate insurance policies for general dentistry. Around 1 million people hold policies that entitle them to register with a private dentist recognised by the insurer. Policies cover both preventive and restorative treatment, and appear to be a direct response to the reduction in the number of dentists willing to do NHS work and the high co-payment for NHS dental treatment
- Norwich Union has entered into an agreement with Medicentres, the walk-in GP clinics, to offer up to four consultations each year (two of which can be substituted with physiotherapy sessions) and GP home visits for a fee of £10 per month.

The dental and GP policies are offered separately from other private medical insurance. Insurance companies told us that they could not combine most primary care services with private medical insurance, because they contained different risks and served distinct audiences. The premiums paid for GP and dental coverage was in the range £10–£15 per month, far less than other individual private medical insurance premiums for elective surgery and the like.

Reviewing insurance policies generally, there is no obvious pattern in the limited and selective cover for extra-hospital services, save that (dentistry excepted) they are limited in comparison with coverage for hospital-based care and the extra-hospital services offered by the NHS. Many of these services have developed as retail markets, and as services covered by health cash plans, with relatively limited involvement from insurers who offer private medical insurance.

Most interestingly for our theme of public–private relations, there are also relatively new forms of private medical insurance policy which cover the costs of private care if people have to wait over a certain period of time for NHS treatment – six weeks in one Norwich Union policy – and pay policyholders a lump sum if they gain access to NHS treatment within the specified period.

Limits to growth in the private medical insurance market

While insurance companies have been successful at creating new products in some areas, progress elsewhere has been limited. For example, the private insurers have straightforward reasons to be interested in general practice. GPs are the gateway to its core secondary care services, but they are a gateway that the private insurers do not control. If they could get a reasonable foothold in general practice, then they could offer vertically integrated services, and so influence referral pathways, among other things, to help keep costs down.

There was considerable insurer interest in general practice in the 1990s. For example in 1994, in the wake of the introduction of the NHS 'internal market', Norwich Union set up a pilot project in a fundholding GP practice in New Milton in Hampshire.[10] The project was 'designed to examine the potential for using private sector techniques in the management of a GP practice fund' rather than directly financing access to general medical services. Norwich Union stated that it was interested in understanding primary care, believing that it would be able to increase its presence over time, and suggesting that it was primarily interested in offering management services rather than extending the private medical insurance market. Presumably, however, expansion of its insurance market also had a place in Norwich Union's thinking. Eventually, the pilot was stopped, partly because GP fundholding was discontinued. When interviewed by us, Norwich Union did not have any pilot schemes running in general practice. As for other private insurers, BUPA also had a pilot scheme in Reading, which it too discontinued. PPP Healthcare currently has a small-scale initiative where people in parts of Dorset are offered the opportunity to sign up with one of six private GPs rather than registering with their usual NHS general practice. Unlike their hospital specialist colleagues, NHS GPs are barred by the terms of their contracts from offering private general medical services to their enrolled NHS patients, so have to offer an entirely separate service if they are to become more than marginally involved in private practice. This severely limits the scope for private provision and insurance in general practice in the UK.

To summarise, the private medical insurance market in the UK is static. Recent attempts to develop the market have generally met with limited success. Insurers face a market that demands more coverage at no greater cost. Given this, it is important to note that the Labour Government explicitly stated in the NHS Plan that private medical insurance will play no part in its plans for health care.[11] The Government argued that private medical insurance was both inefficient and inequitable. Arguments that private insurance may increase welfare in some circumstances (e.g. Besley and Coate[12]) were explicitly rejected. Although it did not say so, it seems that the Government also recognised the practical limits to the use of private medical insurance in the

UK in the face of an NHS. Whether the arguments are about principle or practice, private medical insurance's past appears brighter than its future.

However, it is very unlikely that private medical insurance will disappear entirely. There will continue to be a market for 'double-cover' preferential access to elective specialist treatment, thereby avoiding NHS waiting lists. It seems equally unlikely that low-cost products will disappear, whether modelled on private medical insurance or on health cash plans (see Chapter 3), especially for primary care services such as dentistry and ophthalmic services, for which significant co-payments exist in the NHS.

Private financing: out-of-pocket payment

The other main source of financing for private acute medical care is self-payment. Williams et al.[13] reported that 20.5 per cent of private treatment episodes were self-financed in 1997–98. Our industry respondents pointed out that this was the fastest growing source of finance for private health care. It is covered in greater detail in the next chapter, which focuses on individual forms of payment compared with collective forms of payment for health services.

Private provision: hospitals

Scale

Turning to the provision side of the private market in Table 2.1, Williams et al.[14] reported on the number of patients admitted to private hospitals in England and Wales in 1992–93 and 1997–98 (see Table 2.10). The data show

Table 2.10 Estimated numbers of patients admitted to independent hospitals in England and Wales, 1992–93 and 1997–98*

Year	1992–93	1997–98	Percentage (%) change
Inpatients	429,172	406,843	−5.2
Day cases	249,531	421,580	68.9
Total	678,703	828,422	22.1
Origins of patients			
England and Wales	651,673	805,016	23.5
Other UK	2,556	3,443	34.7
Overseas	20,782	17,199	−17.2
Unknown	3,691	2,764	−

*Adapted from Williams et al. Journal of Public Health Medicine 2000; 22: 68–73.

that over 828,422 people were admitted in 1997–98, split approximately in half between inpatient and day cases. This represented a 22 per cent increase in patient numbers in less than five years. Comparisons with NHS data are not straightforward because data definitions are different in the two sectors, and we do not have separate data for private admissions in Wales. If we assume, though, that the numbers of private patients in Wales is small, and that the data are roughly comparable, then private admissions were around 15 per cent of total admissions for England in 1997–98. This proportion has remained almost constant at this level since 1992–93.

Structure of provision

There are three major independent providers of private hospital services, namely, General Healthcare Group, BUPA and the Nuffield Hospitals Group, which between them have just over half of the market. The rest of the market is divided between half a dozen smaller groups and a larger number of groups with only one or two premises – a number of older charitable hospitals fall into this last group. Most private hospitals are small in relation to NHS general hospitals, typically having 30–50 beds, with 100 beds constituting a large hospital. They provide facilities for a 'core' range of elective procedures, including consulting rooms, day-case suites, operating theatres and inpatient wards.

The sector comprises large numbers of relatively small hospitals. The contrast with the NHS is marked, particularly given the NHS trend towards smaller numbers of ever larger hospitals, driven by a number of factors including reducing lengths of inpatient stay and the perceived value of concentrating resources for major trauma treatment.

It is not difficult to understand why private hospitals are small. One reason is that they undertake a restricted range of procedures. They do not have accident and emergency departments, responsible for about 4 million NHS admissions each year. They need to be located close to their main sources of labour, namely NHS acute hospital trusts. Many clinical staff who do sessions at private hospitals will do most of their work at nearby NHS sites, while others carry out some of their private work in NHS pay beds in NHS hospitals. Thus, private hospitals need to be close enough to make travel distances manageable as they duplicate the elective services provided in the local NHS hospitals. The opportunities to provide a substantial surgical service on any one site are therefore limited.

The small size of hospitals may be one of the causes of the cost-containment problems in the sector, alongside the incentives facing consultants. Economies in the scale of provision must be difficult to achieve for clinical and support staff, and for those facilities and equipment that must be provided on site in any hospital. For example, it is uneconomic to provide a full NHS-style intensive care service in hospitals of 30–50 beds. It must also be difficult in many areas to provide proper medical and nursing cover for post-surgical patients, since the available pool of skilled staff is small, and in most cases substantially committed to the NHS. One might speculate that, in the absence of significant economies of scale, strategies for containing costs may instead have to focus on staffing and facilities.

Three trends in private hospitals

Three trends over the last decade or so are particularly noteworthy. The first is the change in the pattern of services. At one end of the spectrum, there is now far more minimally invasive day surgery than there was at the beginning of the 1990s, while at the other end, there are far more complex neurosurgery, heart surgery and other highly invasive procedures requiring the use of intensive care beds. Some private hospitals now have intensive care beds, though the numbers are low – we estimate that there are fewer than 100 beds in the UK private sector. (Even these, so far as we were able to establish, are staffed and equipped for recovery from surgery, and not for major complications that might arise. Note that providing for surgical recovery alone is less expensive in both capital and revenue terms than providing for any problem that might arise, such as in the case of NHS intensive care units.) A more general indicator of these trends is that while total activity has continued to increase, the number of beds registered with the Department of Health in hospitals and clinics has been falling. The average bed occupancy decreased from 54 per cent in 1990 to around 50 per cent in 1997.[15]

The second trend, discussed above from the insurers' perspective, is that cost pressures within the sector have increased. Laing[16] notes that cost pressures have led both insurers and hospitals to find ways of controlling costs, particularly in the last five years. One development, stimulated by insurers, is towards the identification of selected hospitals that they judge can offer good-quality care at competitive prices. These arrangements tend to favour larger hospital groups that can better afford to monitor the quality of consultants' work, and seems to be leading to reduced use of smaller hospitals, including the few remaining charitable hospitals. This is linked, for some insurers, to the move towards prospective payment for services, where the insurer agrees fixed prices for procedures with hospitals in the network (e.g. diagnosis-related, group-based payments according to a payment schedule).

Hospitals have also developed their own services based on guaranteed fixed prices for selected procedures, some of which they offer directly to patients rather than insurers. In Nuffield Direct, for example, the Nuffield Hospitals group has gone further and offers what are effectively low interest and interest-free loans to enable patients to pay for hospital care by instalments rather than take out insurance. This represents another threat to the private medical insurance market, as well as widening the range of options for the private financing of health care in the UK.

A third trend concerns assurance about the safety and quality of services. The larger groups reported to us that they had increased the resources they devoted to quality assurance in recent years. For aspects of services delivered by their employees, particularly nurses and their general management, they had implemented a number of processes, including the Health Quality Service's organisational audit, and processes based on ISO 9002, an international set of quality standards. (Note that these schemes focus on general organisational processes, and not directly on clinical quality assurance.) Some hospital groups now use patient surveys to establish outcomes and satisfaction for the patients who attend their hospitals. If used properly, these are potentially a powerful source of information about the work of consultants and other health professionals. We were not able, however, to establish the extent to which patient information was used in practice and whether such data would be made available to prospective patients.

BUPA told us that it had been implementing rules that would ensure that surgeons had to undertake reasonable numbers of a particular operation before they could operate in its hospitals. It was also stressed to us that private hospitals were concerned about the possibility of 'another Bristol in one of our hospitals', referring to the tragic case of the heart surgeons who were found guilty of professional misconduct by the General Medical Council in 1998. One might add that it is simply good business practice to offer a good service, and this should not be underestimated as a driver of good-quality care for hospitals and insurers in a competitive market.

Equally, though, some of our hospital-based respondents told us that they had met with relatively limited success in implementing clinical quality assurance processes for consultants. They noted that consultants are independent contractors to private hospital groups, and negotiated with them on a range of matters including clinical quality (as well as costs), but that ultimately hospitals had relatively little control over them. This accords with evidence provided to the Health Committee of the House of Commons from the many individuals and groups reporting bad experiences of using private hospitals. Reflecting on this evidence, the Committee stated that:

> We heard and read graphic and moving evidence of individual tragic cases where patients died in the independent sector. According to relatives of those who died, the deaths occurred as a result of negligence or incompetence. Detailed investigation of the clinical issues to which these relatives drew attention lies beyond the scope of this inquiry, and we are not able to examine individual cases. We do, however, feel it is important to draw attention to those clinical issues which patient representative groups most consistently referred to as contributory factors to additional clinical risk within the independent healthcare sector. These comprised:
>
> - An increased risk to patients occupying single rooms in that they were less well supervised than those in wards.
> - Problems arising from the lack of specialist wards in independent hospitals resulting in less specialised nursing and medical care.
> - Little information available to trusts or private providers as to the overall working hours of staff, resulting in patients being seen by staff who were exhausted.
> - A lack of resuscitation and other emergency back-up facilities.
> - Resident Medical Officers who were inexperienced.
> - An absence of doctors on duty who had taken the Advanced Course in Life Saving Technique.
> - An absence of even informal peer review since clinicians in the independent sector tended not to work in teams as is the case in the NHS.
>
> We have insufficient data to assess how general such problems are in the sector ... Nevertheless the small size of the average private hospital (most have fewer than 100 beds), and the need for it to operate commercially, may jeopardize patient safety.[17]

In the Committee's eyes, hospitals did not always ensure that patients were entering a safe environment, and there must, by extension, be questions about the quality of care they offer. It would be misleading to overstate the problems, and it is important to stress that we were not able to establish their extent, and therefore whether the sector is more or less safer than the NHS for the same procedures. On the other hand, it appears that private insurers and hospital operators, though concerned about quality, currently have limited ability to protect all their patients. The Care Standards Act 2000 is the Government's response to these quality-of-care problems in hospitals and clinics (*see* Chapter 7).

Private provision: consultants and specialists

The practice of hospital consultants in maintaining NHS and private work alongside each other and the problematic implications for the NHS are discussed in Chapter 6. Here, our interest is in the role of hospital specialists while working in the private sector, as the third element of the simple insurer/hospital/consultant framework. Consultants usually work in the private sector as independent contractors, and may see patients in consulting rooms, e.g. in Harley Street, London, or in a hospital. Some two out of three consultants undertake private work, most doing relatively little in relation to their NHS work. BUPA's evidence to the House of Commons Health Committee Inquiry into Consultants' NHS Contracts[18] stated that two-thirds of consultants who work for its hospitals earn less than £10,000 each year. However, a minority earn rather more than that figure, and more data on workload and incomes are presented in Chapter 4.

When consultants work in hospitals, the hospital is, in effect, a provider of facilities and management. Consultants will typically contract to use consulting rooms, operating theatres and other facilities, with the hospital providing these facilities, the nursing and support staff and the management infrastructure that maintains them.

In order to understand the relationships between consultants and hospital groups, it is useful to contrast the situations in the private sector and the NHS. In the NHS, consultants have a team of junior doctors who are there to learn from them and to provide cover when the consultants are not at work. The way in which the NHS system works in practice has both advantages and disadvantages. One disadvantage to NHS patients is that they may be treated by someone with relatively little experience, with some increased clinical risks, as shown by successive reports of the Confidential Inquiry into Perioperative Deaths. An advantage is the fact that you can be treated by a doctor at any time of day or night, because there is always someone on site – even if that person is less experienced than a consultant – and there is consultant back-up when needed. Many NHS hospitals now provide consultant on-site cover round the clock for a range of major specialties.

In private hospitals, consultants do not have junior doctors supporting them. In the nature of private work, most consultants are not on site at a private hospital most of the time. The main commitment for most of them is still to the NHS. There are questions, therefore, about cover when consultants are not on site. We were told that the larger hospital groups have organised round-the-clock cover from surgeons or anaesthetists. For example, all hospitals covered by PPP Healthcare must have on-call medical cover. But adequate cover does not seem to be universal. In some private hospitals, particularly those that are not part of a large chain, we were informed of recent occasions when the on-duty doctor was a GP (i.e. not trained to act in the event of a major complication), providing cover for a hospital in which invasive surgical procedures were routine. This may not be important for minor procedures, when people go home the same day, and for which the proper first action in case of difficulties is to telephone your (NHS-financed) GP. But it clearly does matter with any procedure that requires an inpatient stay because, as discussed above, evidence to the Health Committee of the House of Commons shows that things do go wrong, sometimes seriously.

Some of our industry respondents referred to consultants as their 'business partners', but we gained the impression that consultants held the whip hand in a rather strained relationship. Indeed, it was important for hospitals to keep consultants happy, because without them there would be little or no business. The view was expressed to us that doctors should be able to turn up and get on with their work, in contrast to their NHS roles in which, it was claimed, consultants were far more constrained and had a wider set of responsibilities. In some cases, consultants were also tempted by the opportunity to undertake new procedures, which might not be possible in the NHS, and we heard anecdotal evidence of this happening. This may have important implications for quality and patient protection, particularly if there is relatively little peer supervision in the private sector. We were also told, however, that some hospital groups were now moving towards a more conservative policy, and in the future would only be likely to allow treatments and procedures approved by the National Institute for Clinical Excellence (NICE) for use in the NHS, thus accepting common definitions of appropriateness. As in other instances, we were not able to determine where the truth lay.

The formal relationship between the doctors and the hospital, in all but the smallest hospitals, is between the hospital and its Medical Advisory Committee (MAC). The MAC typically comprises three consultants who work at the hospital. So far as we could establish, consultants control who is on a local MAC. Each hospital has its own MAC, which means that hospital chains have to deal with each hospital in turn. Crucially, in our view, the MAC determines who has admitting rights to the private hospital. The hospital management will, of course, have a view about what sorts of specialists are needed, but it does not directly control who is appointed. In this connection, it is interesting to note the conclusions of the Health Committee.[19] It felt that the accountability of consultants to hospitals and insurers was too weak, and recommended that MACs should be formally responsible – perhaps statutorily responsible – for the quality of clinical care in private hospitals. However, this still omits the supervision of the safety and quality of private care delivered by specialists in their consulting rooms and privately owned clinics (*see* Chapter 3 for a discussion of what can go wrong in private cosmetic surgery clinics).

Private provision: other practitioners

It would be easy to focus entirely on private medical services. But it is important to recognise the wide range of services provided by other practitioners. These include:

- private nursing care provided in hospital, nursing home and domiciliary settings
- professionals allied to medicine, providing therapies such as chiropody and physiotherapy, which have always been available privately
- complementary therapies.

Figure 2.3 indicates the noticeable proportion of nurses who work in private health and social care settings, which is partly due to the move of continuing nursing care out of the NHS in the 1980s.[20,21] Many nurses in the private acute sector are financed through private medical insurance and self-payment channelled into hospitals and clinics. In addition, a substantial amount of private care is provided in residential and nursing homes, and is paid for both by the State (via local authorities) and, in the case of older people, supplemented by individuals from their own savings and their families'. Buchan *et al.*[22] estimated that of the 372,000 whole-time-equivalent registered nurses employed in nursing in 1995, almost 58,000 (15 per cent) worked in private acute or nursing home settings. In a 1998 survey, Smith and

Figure 2.3 Where nurses work

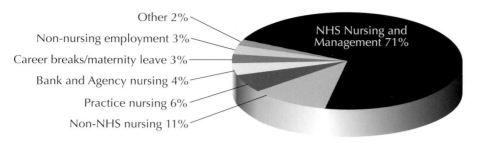

Other 2%
Non-nursing employment 3%
Career breaks/maternity leave 3%
Bank and Agency nursing 4%
Practice nursing 6%
Non-NHS nursing 11%

NHS Nursing and Management 71%

Source: Institute of Employment Studies. *Changing Times: a survey of registered nurses in 1998.* (1998 RCN Membership Survey)

Seccombe[23] estimated that about 11 per cent of nurses worked in non-NHS settings, and a further 4 per cent were bank and agency nurses. Figure 2.2 shows the proportion of nurses in different types of employment.

Some community-based nurses (including the very few private midwives), along with many professionals allied to medicine (e.g. physiotherapists) and almost all complementary therapists, work in what might be called a private retail market. That is, the usual way of paying for a service is directly out-of-pocket. It has been difficult to obtain precise estimates of the extent of private work undertaken by these groups, but indicative data are provided in Chapter 3. It is clear that there are significant markets outside the NHS for a wide range of services.

Some of these services can also be paid for through health cash plans (the insurance products with pre-NHS origins noted earlier). These will be discussed in more detail in Chapter 3, because they are used to pay for services across the NHS–private divide. It should be noted, however, that some of the £250 million per annum of payments made into health cash plans are paid out for claims for private services, including physiotherapy and non-NHS prescriptions for glasses. They are, therefore, another example of private financing and provision of services.

Public financing and private provision

There is also public expenditure on private health services, which takes us into the bottom left quadrant of Table 2.1. Table 2.2 shows that there are some important services in this quadrant. The NHS spent some £50 million on private acute health care contracts in 1998, which is less than 1 per cent of the

NHS budget.[24] Part of this figure can be attributed to the awarding of contracts to the private sector to help reduce NHS waiting times: in 1997–98, the NHS commissioned around 29,000 elective ordinary admissions and 62,000 day cases from the independent sector.[25] Although the current level of services provided in private hospitals for the NHS is small as a proportion of total NHS activity, it is more significant as a proportion of the incomes of private acute hospitals, accounting for over 10 per cent of private acute revenue if abortions are taken into account (*see* Table 2.11). In addition, this proportion may increase in future since the NHS Plan explicitly sanctioned the use of spare capacity in the private sector if this contributed to reducing waiting times for public patients.[26]

Table 2.11 Sources of funding of independent hospitals, residents of England and Wales, 1992–93 and 1997–98*

Source of funding	Patient population, 1992–93	Percentage (%)	Patient population, 1997–98	Percentage (%)
NHS	31,982	4.9	84,561	10.5
Private insured	480,257	73.7	541,111	67.2
Private self-pay	133,567	20.5	165,054	20.5
Private other	37	0.1	9,229	1.1
Not known	5,492	0.8	5,062	0.6
TOTAL	**651,673**	**100.0**	**805,016**	**100.0**

Figures include abortions.
*Adapted from Williams *et al. Journal of Public Health Medicine* 2000; 22: 68–73.

A far more substantial and less well-known area of private provision of publicly financed services is psychiatric care. The 1999 report by the House of Commons Health Committee on the regulation of private health care stated that:

> *The independent sector provides some 67 per cent of beds [used by the NHS] for non-acute psychiatric care in independent nursing homes and residential homes. There is a growing demand for beds for mentally ill and mentally infirm people – the figure for the number of beds in 1998, 25,500, represents an increase of 48 per cent compared with 1994. In acute psychiatry, about 55 per cent of the UK's medium- and low-security beds are provided by the sector. Registered mental nursing home[s] provide over 80 per cent of beds for the care of brain-injured people. About 30 per cent of occupied independent psychiatric beds are funded by the NHS.[27]*

It is important to distinguish here between two policy developments. One of them is the move of continuing nursing care out of the NHS. Changes in rules for social security payments in the early 1980s led to a massive increase in the size of the private nursing and residential home sector.[28] People in this sector have a range of nursing care needs, including those noted by the Health Committee, which the NHS has been reluctant to meet directly. However, the Government's response to the Royal Commission on Long-Term Care[29] has committed the NHS to meeting the nursing component of the care needs of people in both domiciliary and nursing home settings. This is likely to increase the NHS finance of provision that is primarily located in the private sector.

The second, more recent, development is in acute psychiatric care. In the early 1990s, the NHS, particularly in London, found that it did not have enough beds for this group of people. Some health authorities responded by awarding annual contracts to private providers. This extra-contractual referral mechanism was also used to admit people to private psychiatric beds. It appears that the demise of extra-contractual referrals, with the abolition of the internal market in 1997–98, has not led to a reduction in the use of private beds. Rather, a new balance has been created by which the NHS uses its funds to purchase beds from the private sector. This development has occurred with relatively little comment, despite the scale of the shift of provision into the private sector by the NHS.

It is also important to note the role of the voluntary (or 'third') sector in providing some types of care. Again, to quote the Health Committee report:

> The NHS makes significant use of the voluntary sector to provide palliative care. Of the 171 hospice units in England, 35 are run by the NHS which manages only 17.5 per cent of all specialist palliative care beds in England.[30]

Private finance and public provision

The final quadrant in Table 2.1 relates to private finance and public provision. Many readers will be surprised that there is anything in this quadrant at all: the notion that there should be private financing of the NHS seems odd given that the NHS is often regarded as the archetypal, monolithic, publicly financed, health system. In fact, there are two important examples. The first of these is NHS pay beds, which were part of the 1946 Settlement between the Government and the medical profession. These are beds in NHS hospitals which consultants can use for their private patients, with the income going to the hospital and the specialist in the form of fees. Laing estimates that about 40 per cent of NHS private patient income is funded through private medical insurance, as opposed to 70 per cent for private hospitals, with the balance coming from self-payment.

Pay beds are of three main types. The first is located in dedicated pay bed units. There are some 1375 beds in 75 pay bed units, which are not generally used by NHS patients. In 1994–95, the last year for which data are available, there were 99,399 admissions to pay bed units.[31] The total of ordinary and day case admissions to NHS hospitals was 4,061,197, making pay bed admissions just under 2.4 per cent of all NHS admissions.[32] The total income of these units was over £250 million in 1997, which represents 16 per cent of the private acute hospital market.[33] Thus, the NHS is a significant provider (as well as purchaser) in the private acute hospital sector, and has a similar 'market share' to the large private providers such as BUPA hospitals.

The second type of NHS pay bed is dispersed throughout general NHS hospital wards. These are beds for which private patients have priority. Their formal status is not the same as beds in dedicated pay bed units, since they are used by NHS patients if there is no private patient present to use them. There are about 1600 of these beds across the NHS, and there are no reliable figures for their utilisation, though Laing[34] estimates that occupancy of these beds by private patients may be as low as 10 per cent.

The third type of unit is operated by private firms on NHS sites. These appeared in the early 1990s. These are effectively independent hospitals built on NHS land. The main links with the NHS hospitals will be a lease for the site, some sharing of supplies' purchasing, and contracts for the use of facilities, such as scanners in the NHS hospital, by private patients. Data are not available for the income or activity of these units, though there are only a handful of such units.

This quadrant of Table 2.1 also contains user charges for NHS services, including non-hospital dentistry, GP drug prescriptions and NHS eyesight tests, which totalled £800 million in 1998, or about 2 per cent of the NHS budget.[35] These are services that were free at the founding of the NHS. However, GP prescription and non-hospital dental charges were introduced in 1951. (Complex non-hospital dental procedures had had to be paid for from the start of the NHS in 1948.) Over and above the charges, there have been changes in the patterns of provision of general dental services. Hayward[36] reports that the proportion of general dentistry provided privately rose from 5 per cent of treatments in 1992–93 to 25 per cent in 1996–97, partly, and significantly, because the 1992 general dental contract proved to be financially unattractive to many dentists.

As with dentistry, there have been significant changes in the public–private mix of people having eyesight tests. Following the abolition of free NHS eyesight tests in 1989, most adults had to pay for them, with about half of all NHS eyesight tests being carried out without charge, while the other half attracted user charges. The balance then changed again after the Labour Government restored free eyesight tests for people aged 60 years and over from April 1999 (*see* Figure 2.4), with free NHS tests probably now accounting for over 60 per cent of tests. Propper[37] has derived figures from the British Household Panel survey, which illustrates the extent of private uptake of selected primary care services and tracks these shifts in NHS support (*see* Table 2.12).

There are other items in the private finance and public provision quadrant of **Figure 2.4** NHS sight tests paid for by FHSAs/HAs*[1]

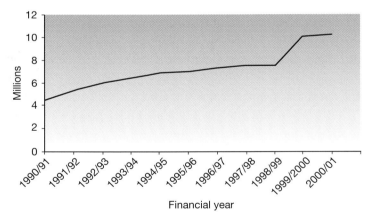

Financial year

1. Eligibility to NHS sight tests was extended to all patients aged 60 and over from 1 April 1999.
*Source: Department of Health. *General Ophthalmic Services Activities Statistics, April – December 2000*, 2001.

Table 2.1. One item relates to the Labour Government's recent announcement that it will formalise the requirement for car insurers to meet the costs of NHS treatment relating to road accidents. Another is the use of National Lottery funding – which originates from individuals' pockets after tax – for the NHS. Private individuals also fund the NHS directly through charitable giving (*see*

Table 2.12 Private health care services as percentage of total UK health care expenditure in British Household Panel survey*

Service	1990–91	1991–92	1992–93	1993–94	1994–95
Dental care	9.0	8.5	N/A	11.6	12.7
Eye care	8.6	8.4	10.5	10.0	10.7
Physiotherapy, chiropody and health visitor	4.0	4.2	4.9	5.2	5.0

*Adapted from Propper. *The Demand for Private Health Care in the UK,* 1999.

Chapter 3). This quadrant, while small in money terms relative to some of the others, is nevertheless rather larger than might have been expected.

Conclusion

The data presented in this chapter have been organised to highlight the permutations of public and private finance, and public and private provision of services present in UK health care. The descriptive material demonstrates the continuing dominance of the NHS both in finance and provision, but coupled with substantial expenditure and activity outside the NHS, as well as private sources of funding and activity within the NHS. Table 2.11 highlights this complexity by providing estimates for the different sources of financing of private hospital care. The NHS, as already noted, is a significant financier of private hospitals.

The UK is currently positioned between countries such as Norway, where the State finances almost all health care, and many other OECD countries, where private contributions are in the range of 20–25 per cent of total spending.[38] Since 1980, there has been a gradual increase in the share of private funding of health care in the UK. It is sufficiently large for its effects to need to be taken into account in health policy-making in the UK. This is especially so given the extent of private finance and activity within the NHS and the possible impact of the private sector on the working of the NHS. As we shall see in later chapters, the current pattern of private finance and provision poses questions for equity and for consumer protection in UK health care.

References

1 Salter B. *The Politics of Change in the Health Service*. Basingstoke: Macmillan, 1998.
2 Propper C. Who pays for and who gets health care? *Equity in the Finance and Delivery of Health Care in the United Kingdom*. Nuffield Occasional Papers Health Economics Series: Paper #5. London: Nuffield Trust, 1998.

3   *OECD Health Data* CD Rom. Paris: OECD, 2001.

4   Laing and Buisson. *Laing's Healthcare Market Review 1999–2000*. London: Laing and Buisson, 1999.

5   Association of British Insurers. *Data Briefing*. London: ABI, 1998.

6   Laing and Buisson. *Laing's Healthcare Market Review 1999–2000*. London: Laing and Buisson, 1999.

7   Office for National Statistics. *Social Trends 29*. London: Stationery Office, 1999: 140.

8   Laing and Buisson. *Laing's Healthcare Market Review 1999–2000*. London: Laing and Buisson, 1999.

9   Ibid.

10 Norwich Union. *Into the Future: developing primary care organisations*. Eastleigh: Norwich Union Healthcare, 1996.

11 Secretary of State for Health. *The NHS Plan: a plan for investment; a plan for reform*. Cm 4818-I. London: Stationery Office, 2000: 33.

12 Besley T, Coate S. Public provision of private goods and the redistribution of income. *American Economic Review* 1991; 81: 979–84.

13 Williams B, Rushton L, Whatmough P, McGill J. Patients and procedures in short-stay independent hospitals in England and Wales, 1997–1998. *Journal of Public Health Medicine* 2000; 22: 68–73.

14 Ibid.

15 Department of Health. *Private Hospitals, Homes and Clinics*. Statistical Bulletin 1998/14.

16 Laing and Buisson. *Laing's Healthcare Market Review 1999–2000*. London: Laing and Buisson, 1999.

17 Health Committee. *The Regulation of Private and Other Independent Healthcare*. Volume I. London: Stationery Office, 1999.

18 BUPA. *Focusing on Health Benefits. Written evidence to the House of Commons Health Committee Inquiry into Consultants' NHS Contracts*. London: BUPA, 2000.

19 Health Committee. *The Regulation of Private and Other Independent Healthcare*. Volume I. London: Stationery Office, 1999.

20 Pollock A. The NHS goes private. *Lancet* 1995; 346: 683–4.

21 Royal Commission on Long-Term Care. *With Respect to Old Age*. Cm 4192-I. London: Stationery Office, 1999.

22 Buchan J, Seccombe I, Smith G. *Nurses Work: an analysis of the UK nursing labour market*. Aldershot: Ashgate, 1998.

23 Smith G, Seccombe I. *Changing Times: a survey of registered nurses in 1998*. Brighton: Institute for Employment Studies, 1998.

24 Laing and Buisson. *Laing's Healthcare Market Review 1999–2000*. London: Laing and Buisson, 1999.

25 Department of Health. *Private Hospitals, Homes and Clinics*. Statistical Bulletin 1998/14.

26 Secretary of State for Health. *The NHS Plan: a plan for investment; a plan for reform*. Cm 4818-I. London: Stationery Office, 2000: 97–8.

27 Health Committee. *The Regulation of Private and Other Independent Healthcare*. Volume I. London: Stationery Office, 1999.

28 Sinclair I, Parker R, Leat D, Williams J. *The Kaleidoscope of Care*. London: HMSO, 1990.

29 Secretary of State for Health. *The NHS Plan. The Government's response to the Royal Commission on Long-Term Care*. Cm 4818-II. London: Stationery Office, 2000.

30 Health Committee. *The Regulation of Private and Other Independent Healthcare*. Volume I. London: Stationery Office, 1999.

31 Williams B. Utilisation of National Health Service hospitals in England by private patients 1989–95. *Health Trends* 1997; 29: 21–5.

32 Health Committee. *Public Expenditure on Health and Personal Social Services 1998*. HC 959, Session 1997–98. London: Stationery Office, 1998.

33 Laing and Buisson. *Laing's Healthcare Market Review 1999–2000*. London: Laing and Buisson, 2000.

34 Ibid.

35 Department of Health. *Departmental Report 2000*. London: Stationery Office, 2000.

36 Hayward J. NHS dentistry. In: Harrison A, editor. *Health Care UK 1998–99*. London: King's Fund, 1999.

37 Propper C. *The Demand for Private Health Care in the UK*. Centre for Markets and Public Organisation working paper. Bristol: University of Bristol, October 1999.

38 *OECD Health Data*. CD Rom. Paris: OECD, 2001.

Chapter 3

Individual versus collective payment in the UK

Introduction

In Chapter 2, the relations between public and private health services were mapped in terms of a reasonably conventional distinction between public and private finance, and public and private provision. However, a different, less conventional way of thinking about the financing of health care in public and private sectors is in terms of who pays. Much of the finance described in Chapter 2 came from 'collective' sources in both public and private spheres, namely the State and private insurance companies, i.e. there is risk-pooling. This arrangement can be contrasted with individual full payment, or co-payment, for a specific service, whereby people pay for what they need at the time they need it, and the transaction has the general features of a retail purchase, i.e. no risk-pooling. Table 3.1, which is a variant of Table 2.1 in Chapter 2, distinguishes between individual and collective payments for health care.

Table 3.1 Individual and collective financing of health care

	Individual financing from after-tax income	Collective financing
Public provision of services	Co-payments for NHS services (e.g. dentistry, eyesight tests) funded by cash payments or using health cash plans	NHS
Private provision of services	Cash payments	Private medical insurance policies, health cash plans used for private services

We described in some detail the nature and scale of collective payments in Chapter 2, particularly private medical insurance, and so focus in this chapter on individual payments. Just as UK policy debates often omit private medical insurance and private acute provision, so they also tend to leave out any discussion of products and services funded directly by individuals, especially outside the NHS. Private medical insurance providers are increasingly having to compete with the attractions of self-insurance as people make use of their savings and current income to pay for private care directly. As we will see, this type of expenditure is far from negligible, though it can be difficult to quantify. We then turn to other forms of payment for health care, such as health cash plans that are designed to enable people to pay for care out-of-pocket. We end by discussing the overall balance of individual and collective payments in the UK.

In principle, individual payments can have both positive and negative effects for patients in terms of consumer protection and equity. One positive argument is that individuals can make (reasonably) informed and affordable choices about some straightforward, low-cost health products, such as cold remedies or sticking plasters, and should therefore be able to do so. The clinical risks associated with their use are judged to be low (by the State and by many consumers), and the creation of markets has led to those products being provided at competitive prices. Market prices for some products and services may also discourage 'frivolous' demand, though it is difficult to be sure how strong this argument is in practice. Less positively, charging or part-charging, even for basic health care services, tends to increase inequities in the financing and use of health care, since people on average and below-average incomes may not be able to afford them easily, or at all.[1]

In this chapter, we discuss five domains of individual payment in the UK, namely:

- over-the-counter medicines and other retail health care products
- out-of-pocket payments for private surgical services
- out-of-pocket payment for private non-surgical services, such as those provided by physiotherapists, other clinical professionals and complementary therapists (the services of the last group are mostly not paid for, or provided, by the NHS)
- other forms of individual payment
- out-of-pocket payment for NHS services.

Figure 3.1 provides the financial context for the discussion. The Office for National Statistics (ONS) estimated non-NHS health care expenditure at just over £8 billion in 1997 (about 16 per cent of total health care spending). In the same period, about £2.1 billion was spent on insurance, by private

Figure 3.1 Estimated individual financing of health care

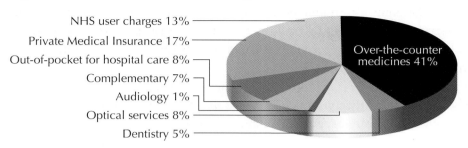

NHS user charges 13%
Private Medical Insurance 17%
Out-of-pocket for hospital care 8%
Complementary 7%
Audiology 1%
Optical services 8%
Dentistry 5%
Over-the-counter medicines 41%

individuals and by companies on behalf of their employees, as noted in Chapter 2.

Thus, there is about £6 billion of non-NHS health care expenditure to be accounted for: Figure 3.1 shows our estimated breakdown of this amount. Data on these payments are collected from a variety of sources, sometimes from solid data and at other times from the best available estimates. The payments appear to fall into three broad categories. The first category involves payments made out-of-pocket. According to ONS, just under £2.5 billion was spent on pharmaceuticals in 1997. This amount is larger than the £1.47 billion reported in the research literature as spent on over-the-counter medicines in the same year.[2,3,4] The ONS amount refers only to pharmaceuticals – and not, for example, to any lifestyle products – and is the amount used in Figure 3.1. This category also includes private payment for dentistry (over £300 million) and optical services (about £480 million). Optical services include eyesight tests and spectacle and contact lens prescriptions. Dentistry and optical services are discussed in Chapter 4.

Payment for complementary therapies, such as osteopathy and acupuncture, is at least £450 million per year according to research by Kate Thomas of the University of Sheffield (personal communication), and has been estimated at £500 million by the House of Lords Science and Technology Committee.[5] Private individuals pay £500 million each year directly out-of-pocket on hospital treatment. Self-payment has been growing in recent years, and about 20 per cent of procedures are now paid for directly rather than through insurance.

Some commentators would add long-term care to the self-payment category. Figures for personal health care expenditure of people living in their own homes or living in nursing or residential homes are difficult to establish, but estimates prepared for the Royal Commission on Long-Term Care[6] suggest that expenditure runs into hundreds of millions of pounds. Private expenditure on chiropody alone is about £70 million each year. These figures are not included in Figure 3.1, but only because we could not obtain reliable estimates for all the relevant services involved.

The second category consists of payments made to third parties that find their way into health care expenditure. These include charitable donations, which total over £150 million each year to the NHS, according to a recent National Audit Office (NAO) report,[7] and National Lottery contributions to the NHS, currently running at £56 million per year.[8] (The latter is not included in Figure 3.1, having started after 1997.)

The third category of individual payment is directly to the NHS. The slogan that the NHS is 'free at the point of delivery' has never been entirely accurate, and since 1951 patients have had to pay user charges. Today, the bulk of charges are for prescriptions, dentistry and ophthalmic services, and totalled £800 million in 1997–98.[9]

Another way of looking at spending by individuals is using surveys of all household expenditure. Table 3.2 shows the amounts spent by households in each income decile on basic health care products including medicines and plasters, and paid-for services, which rises from under £1 per week (i.e. about £50 each year) for the lowest income decile, to about £5 per week for the highest decile.

Retail payment

A substantial volume of health care is dealt with outside the boundaries of formal health services. A key instance is private individuals purchasing products from a pharmacy (partly straddling the formal health service and retail sectors), supermarket or other outlet. The market comprises many different products, but the major products in terms of sales included pain relievers, skin treatments (e.g. Savlon, Zovirax cream) and cold remedies.[10] This market has been growing steadily for many years, and seems likely to go on growing in coming years, partly because of a trend for some formerly prescription-only drugs to be made available either over the counter or via 'pharmacist-only' sale. This shift away from drugs subsidised by the NHS with a flat-rate user charge, and the wide range of exemptions to retail sale with no subsidy, greatly increases the number of people having to pay the full cost of a

Table 3.2 Detailed household expenditure by gross income decile group, 1997–98*

	Lowest ten per cent	Second decile group	Third decile group	Fourth decile group	Fifth decile group	Sixth decile group	Seventh decile group	Eighth decile group	Ninth decile group	Highest ten per cent	All households
Medicines, prescriptions, spectacles	0.6	1.1	1.3	1.7	1.9	3.9	3.3	3.1	3.4	4.5	2.5
Medical, dental, optical and nursing fees	0.3	0.3	0.6	1.3	1.0	1.3	1.5	1.9	1.5	3.9	1.4
Total	**0.9**	**1.4**	**1.9**	**3.0**	**2.9**	**5.2**	**4.8**	**5.0**	**4.9**	**8.4**	**3.9**

*Adapted from Office for National Statistics. *Consumer Trends*, 1999.

pharmaceutical. This is likely to have a generally regressive effect, since those with the highest need for such items are likely to be on lower incomes.

Large private firms have a long-standing presence in this primary care market in the UK. The most interesting single company is Boots, a presence on many UK high streets. For decades now, Boots has had a substantial share of the prescription drug and over-the counter pharmaceutical markets. It now also offers complementary medicines. In recent years, it has added a chain of opticians, and is now one of the four large-scale optician chains across the UK. More recently, it has started to offer a primary dental service, whereby adults can have a fixed-price private treatment session (the service is not offered to children). Boots also offers influenza vaccinations for about £20.

The move of Boots into dentistry has been matched by a number of other large firms that now own 'dental bodies corporate'. These are legal entities that allow for the provision of salaried private dental services. In effect, they are an alternative organisational structure to the NHS. Having attracted little corporate interest until recently, they are now being used to create chains of dental services, broadly in line with the model that has developed in optical services.

Boots pre-eminently, but accompanied by other corporations, have therefore developed into providers of a wide range of primary health care goods and services. We were told by respondents working in the retail sector that there is considerable competition in the over-the-counter market, and increasingly in the prescription market, stimulated in large part by the entry of the major supermarket chains. Thus, increased competition has provided firms such as Boots with incentives to diversify into new markets. Indeed, Boots also now offers a health cash plan, so it is also diversifying into health care financing.

It is difficult to judge how well the structure of the markets for these goods and services serves the interests of consumers. For the most part, the goods and services involved carry low clinical risks, and competition will tend to improve their value for money. For us, the important point is that large private firms are expanding across a range of primary care services. As we will argue in Chapter 7, it is time for a review of such developments to ensure that the interests of consumers are protected.

Out-of-pocket payment for private surgical services

General elective surgery

Approximately 20 per cent of private acute hospital health care, or £0.5 billion per annum, is paid for directly by individuals. The proportion paid for directly has increased from about 12 per cent in 1992–93. The reasons why this percentage has increased are not clear, but a combination of factors was suggested by some of our interviewees. On the 'supply side', there has been a general increase in disposable income, particularly among older working adults, and people with money in savings are able to use their savings for operations, if needed. On the 'demand side', NHS waiting lists and waiting times were on the increase until 1997, so that people who did not have private medical insurance and were not content to wait might have paid for operations out of their own pockets. It was also suggested that more people were deciding that private medical insurance policies, which have been increasing in price in real terms, no longer represented such good value for money.

On this last point, the OFT has published a useful table of the expected value of the 'non-core' benefits of private medical insurance products (Table 3.3). OFT's purpose was to show how different policies could be compared. OFT has identified services covered by some private medical insurance policies, but not others, and the marginal price of covering them. Table 3.3 suggests that the 'return' on private medical insurance premiums is low for some conditions – it would be interesting to see the results of more detailed actuarial work on the value of private medical insurance premiums.

Further stimulating the market for out-of-pocket payment for surgery, private hospital operators are increasingly interested in helping patients finance their operations directly without private medical insurance. Nuffield Hospitals have developed Nuffield Direct, a finance plan enabling patients to borrow money for surgery and pay for it by instalments at competitive interest rates.

Table 3.3 Estimate of 'non-core' benefits of private medical insurance policies*

Benefit	Average cost of each episode (£)	Likely annual frequency	Estimated annual benefit (£)
Hospital stay – extra coverage	500	0.02	10.00
Outpatient services	60	0.75	4.50
Parental accommodation	100	0.001	0.10

*Adapted from Office of Fair Trading. *Health Insurance*, 1996.

Cosmetic surgery

Another important focus of out-of-pocket payment is cosmetic surgery, since it is not covered by private medical insurance due to its discretionary nature. The 20 per cent of privately financed hospital care paid for out-of-pocket by individuals includes little cosmetic surgery, since it tends to be provided in small specialist clinics rather than private hospitals. Cosmetic surgery has attracted attention both because of the damage that has been done to people by some surgeons, which can be all too visible, and because it is expensive and yet has to be paid for out-of-pocket.

The NHS offers little discretionary cosmetic surgery, such as breast or nose modifications, so that those who want these procedures must use a private service for which they pay directly. In contrast to the other retail goods and services discussed above, the price of surgery is typically counted in thousands of pounds rather than tens.

In its report on the regulation of private health care, the Health Committee of the House of Commons[11] noted that it is common practice to insist on full payment before cosmetic surgery, so that individuals are exposing themselves to both clinical and financial risks. The Committee noted that:

> Advertising clearly plays a considerable part in persuading men and women to consider undergoing cosmetic surgery and other similar treatments. Those individuals are then placed in environments which lack many of the safeguards patients might find elsewhere in the NHS and in the independent sector. They are nearly always self-funded, so there is no medical insurer offering some degree of oversight of activities. They are often self-referred, so there is no GP advising them on where to go for treatment, or indeed on the appropriateness of treatment. On arrival at the clinic, or in preliminary telephone discussions, they are often interviewed by medically unqualified sales consultants, who may be acting on commission.[12]

There is no formal surgical qualification to undertake cosmetic surgery in the UK, so that while some surgeons undoubtedly have appropriate skills, the evidence is that others clearly do not. There are many accounts from individuals who were operated on by someone without appropriate surgical training, where the surgery went wrong, leaving them with serious operation scars, rather than the improved noses or breasts they wanted. The lack of recognised surgical qualifications for cosmetic surgery, the custom of requiring up-front payment, the delivery of the service in small clinics which are not inspected in the same manner as private hospitals and the absence of third-party payer oversight from an insurer, together point to an increased risk for patients. Provisions in the Care Standards Act 2000 may lead to strengthening of consumer protection in this area, as discussed in Chapter 7.

Out-of-pocket payment for private non-surgical services

Private nursing services

Nurses work in the NHS, private health care and social care settings. Even where nurses work outside the NHS, many of the services they provide are paid for by the State (including local authority funding of social care services) or through private medical insurance. But about 20 per cent of their services are paid for directly by individuals. As a result, some acute nursing care is paid for out-of-pocket.

Private general practitioner services

The vast majority of general practice is provided in the NHS, and as far as we are able to judge only 200 GPs operate exclusively in the private sector in England, concentrated in London. However, there have been recent attempts to set up private GP services separate from the NHS. An interesting recent example is Medicentres, which offers a private walk-in GP service. These are services based in busy areas, such as mainline railway stations (particularly in London) and shopping centres. For a fixed fee of about £35, a GP will see people at a time of their choosing, at least during working hours. There are also GP visiting services within a small radius of some of the centres, but the basic service is the walk-in clinic. From their own literature, it is evident that Medicentres are explicitly designed for people who cannot easily arrange to see their own GP, perhaps because they have busy working lives. Or, conversely, GPs are not adjusting their hours to suit modern working practices.

Medicentres attracted a great deal of publicity during 1998 and in the first half of 1999, even though there were never more than 12 of them. However, the column inches did not reflect growth in the service, and while the company that ran them made an operating profit in 1998–99, growth was slower than originally hoped, and Medicentres was sold to another group.

Services of professions allied to medicine

A number of other private clinical services, including physiotherapy and chiropody, are well established. These tend to be overlooked. Even when policy discussions turn to private health care, private doctors tend to dominate. On the other hand, we were unable to identify reliable figures for the extent of private work undertaken by professionals allied to medicine, such as chiropodists and physiotherapists, except for the amount quoted above for chiropody provided in the context of long-term care. The only other evidence about private work comes indirectly from the evidence provided to NHS pay review bodies, as shown in Table 3.4. This shows that the number of professionals leaving the NHS for private work formed a significant proportion of those leaving the NHS. Similarly, the number of professionals leaving training schools in 1996 was 3498, of whom only 850 (24.3 per cent) joined the NHS.[13] Of course, some of the remainder may not have started work. Nevertheless, the figures for leavers and new recruits taken together suggest a substantial private sector for professionals allied to medicine. The numbers either not joining the NHS or leaving it are startling and suggest a problem in the making for the NHS if it wants to be able to continue to provide such services itself. The NHS needs to monitor the situation carefully and understand what is driving employment choices among professionals allied to medicine.

Table 3.4 Professions allied to medicine: leaving the NHS to work outside*†

Year	Total leavers from NHS employment	Leaving the NHS to employment outside	Percentage (%) of total
1991–92	3028	871	28.8
1992–93	2808	745	26.5
1993–94	2339	985	42.1
1994–95	2481	1052	42.4
1995–96	2223	1961	88.2
1996–97	2003	1735	86.6

*Adapted from Chartered Society of Physiotherapy. *Staff Side Evidence 1998,* 1998: 31.
†Professionals allied to medicine defined as including art and music therapy, chiropody, dietetics, occupational therapy, orthoptics, physiotherapy, radiography; total professionals allied to medicine workforce in 1996 estimated at 68,000, about 1 in 3 working part time, 42,850 whole time equivalents.

Complementary therapies

A wide range of complementary therapies is offered privately in the UK. Although different definitions of complementary therapies have been devised, information on numbers of professionals, treatments, expenditure and so on is generally only available for the best established services, such as osteopathy, chiropractic, treatment using herbal medicine, homoeopathy, acupuncture and hypnotherapy. In 1993, Thomas and colleagues[14] estimated that about one in ten people in the UK had used one of these six therapies in the previous 12 months, and that almost 25 per cent had used a herbal, homoeopathic or dietary supplement bought over the counter.

The market for complementary therapies has grown substantially over the last ten years or so, though it is difficult to quantify the growth or the current total size of the market. The House of Lords Science and Technology Committee inquiry into complementary therapies[15] estimated the market at £500 million per annum, but if anything this underestimates the total size of the market. A small proportion (about 5 per cent) of the main complementary therapies is available on the NHS, while osteopathy and homoeopathy are covered by some health cash plans (*see below*). However, the majority of therapies are provided on the basis of payment per session.

There are some data that suggest the scale of individual complementary therapies, though if anything this tends to confuse the picture. For example, the number of chiropractors in the UK is currently about 1200 and they treat approximately 90,000 patient sessions each week (or more than 4.5 million patient sessions each year). If the average payment per patient session is £30, then this implies a total payment of about £140 million per annum for chiropractic. Although the NHS–private split for this therapy is not known precisely, more than 95 per cent of chiropractic is estimated to be private work. Similar data for other therapies are not available. However, the uptake of therapies is believed to have increased greatly over the last five years. Evidence supporting this belief includes increases in the numbers of practitioners. For example, the number of acupuncturists registered with a professional body rose from 507 in 1991 to 3700 in 1997.[16] Retail complementary medicines are now widely available in high street chemists, as well as in health food stores, where they have traditionally been sold, and their use seems certain to have increased.

The situation is complicated by the fact that complementary therapies are sometimes paid for by the NHS, following referrals from GPs or consultants. In 1995, Thomas *et al.*[17] estimated that 45 per cent of NHS GPs recommend or endorse the use of complementary therapy in an average week, 21 per cent refer a patient for complementary therapy (private or NHS) and 10 per cent treat a patient with one of the therapies listed above. They found that 6 per cent of NHS general practices had a complementary health care practitioner working on the premises. Twenty-one per cent of practices reported having a member of the primary health care team who could provide a complementary therapy, and 25 per cent of practices reported making NHS referrals for complementary therapies.

We found it difficult to establish the ways in which individuals generally find and access complementary therapy practitioners. We were told that word of mouth plays an important role, and GPs may recommend a practitioner even if they cannot refer someone as an NHS patient. It was also difficult to assess how well the way in which complementary therapy services are organised protects consumer interests. There is clearly a large constituency that supports complementary medicine, and also evidence that certain procedures can be beneficial. However, we could not find any reliable evidence to prove the safety and quality of UK practice. In light of the growth of complementary medicine, it seems that the ways in which it is accessed, and consumer perceptions of safety, quality and value for money, would be fruitful areas for study.

Other forms of individual payment

Health cash plans

Another source of out-of-pocket payments is health cash plans. They are a form of not-for-profit insurance, though they work along different lines to private medical insurance since they are designed simply to provide cash that patients can use to settle their health care bills directly. They are, strictly, a form of risk-pooling but they are discussed in the context of individual payments because they are designed to enable individual retail payment for services. Note that contributions to health cash plans, and charitable donations which are discussed below, are not included in Figure 3.1. In the case of health cash plans, this is done principally to avoid double-counting, as the plans are used to pay for optical and dental services, among other services.

Health cash plans are used to defray the costs of a wide range of services. Historically, health cash plans were designed to offset the costs associated with going into hospital before the NHS came into being, but today they typically provide a mix of lump sums and weekly payments for a range of other services, including dental services, optical services and physiotherapy. When you use a service that is covered by the plan, you make a claim for reimbursement from the company, who will then send you a cheque. This means that there is no direct link between the plan and the provider of the service, while the sum paid by the plan is fixed, irrespective of the actual cost of the service (unlike under private medical insurance). Indeed, it does not matter who provides the treatment, and payment may be made whether a service is provided privately or by the NHS. Table 3.5 shows an example of costs associated with plans that cover both types of service.

The markets for health cash plans and private medical insurance have been separate for most of their histories. While both are insurance products, they work in different ways. Health cash plans are offered by mutual organisations, and in practice today almost all of them form a special class of mutual organisation, known as friendly societies. They are not-for-profit organisations owned by their members. Premium payments are typically made weekly, for periods of a year at a time, to cover individuals or whole families. Coverage is typically only for people aged between 18 and 64 years, though some plans cover people up to 70 or 74 years of age. The amount of cash paid can be small, starting at under £1 per week. There is also a market in company health cash plans, and some large firms such as Marks and Spencer and British Telecom offer plans to their workforces. (Note that the same firms provide private medical insurance as a benefit only to senior staff.) Unlike private medical insurance, however, the payments made are fixed, and may or may not cover the actual cost of treatment.

There has been substantial growth in the health cash market in recent years, to the point where it is estimated at £200 million to £250 million per annum. This is far smaller than the private medical insurance market, but, unlike private medical insurance, is growing rather than remaining static.[18] Furthermore, there are new entrants into the market. For example, Boots, the high street pharmacy and retail chain, offers a product that gives cash lump sums for dentistry, optical services, physiotherapy, chiropody and other locally provided services. In addition, Abbey National offers a similar product, as does BUPA. The logic behind the entry of new suppliers into the market appears simple: health cash plans are fairly easy for people to understand, and the application forms can be filled in easily. Boots has a large distribution network (as does Abbey National), with large numbers of potential customers using its stores every day. It is unclear how well they are doing, or whether other retail companies will also offer similar plans in the future. However, these plans do offer access to financial help with the costs of private, mostly primary care, services to a wider range of people than is covered by private medical insurance.

Table 3.5 HSA 'Crown Plan': examples of benefits

Weekly payment	Dental care*	Optical care*	Chiropody	Hearing aid	Hospital inpatient	Accident casualty admission	Home help	Mental health treatment
Coverage	Family	Family	Family	Family	Member and partner	Member and partner	Family	Member and partner
£2.40	Up to £60 each	Up to £56 each	Up to £50 each	Up to £40 each	£18 each per night	£18 each per night	Up to £280 per year	£18 per night†
£7.20	Up to £180 each	Up to £168 each	Up to £150 each	Up to £120 each	£54 each per night	£54 each per night	Up to £840 per year	£54 per night

*Benefit of half the amount paid to the dentist or optician.
†20 nights or less – lump sum of £380 for longer stays.

Charitable donations

There are additional individual payments that are rarely noted. The brief history of public–private relations given in Chapter 1 outlined the role of charitable donations in funding voluntary hospitals before the foundation of the NHS. Charitable donations still continue, though now directly to the NHS, and have been estimated at between £469 million and £563 million in 1994–95.[19] A more recent National Audit Office (NAO) report has suggested that annual contributions amounted to £189 million in 1998–99. Almost all of this money was used to fund investments in buildings and equipment rather than staff costs, all items that the NHS itself would otherwise have had to fund. There is also considerable investment income from past bequests, which takes the total Trust income to about £350 million.[20] In addition to this charitable giving, Lottery money is a new source of finance for the NHS, currently £50 million each year. Private health care providers also receive charitable donations, particularly to hospices, but we were unable to obtain data on the amounts.

Out-of-pocket payment for NHS services

The income to the NHS from user charges for GP-prescribed pharmaceuticals, ophthalmic services and dentistry is now £800 million, which equates to 2 per cent of the total NHS budget.[21] The charges are applied in different ways for these services. Generally speaking, for GP prescriptions, people are either exempt from payments, e.g. if they are under 16 years of age, or are liable to pay a fixed sum per item, i.e. they make a co-payment to the NHS.

NHS dentistry is also funded through co-payments, with individuals currently paying on average 80 per cent of the costs of treatment through a tariff of charges covering 400 different procedures. About 20 per cent of all general (non-hospital) dentistry is now entirely financed privately. A proportion of this will be paid for through dental insurance or health cash plans. But many routine visits to the dentist cost in the region of £20–£30, and are paid for out-of-pocket. We were not able to find estimates for the balance between payment from insurance and direct payment.

Until 1989, eyesight tests were free on the NHS, but since then nearly half of adults and older people have had to pay for them, so that 53 per cent (or 8.1 million tests) were provided free and 47 per cent (7.1 million) were paid for privately by individuals in 1998.[22] Private tests cost on average about £18. People who need prescriptions for spectacles may be eligible for vouchers – this applies to children under 16 years of age, and people claiming certain benefits, but not older people. People who are eligible receive vouchers, with the value of the voucher varying according to the nature of their eyesight problem. Over half of people who use vouchers choose to spend an amount greater than the voucher value on their spectacles, paying the difference from their own pockets.[23] People who are not eligible have to pay for spectacles themselves.

The income from NHS user charges grew in the 1980s under successive Conservative administrations, but the Labour Government has indicated that it wishes to slow the rate of increase in charges, and extend free coverage to new groups of patients in the case of GP prescriptions. In the 1998 Budget, the Chancellor of the Exchequer announced that free eyesight tests would be restored to people over 60 years of age from April 2000. The Government has not, however, suggested that it will abolish user charges, and indeed it increased GP prescription charges from £5.80 in 1998 to £6.10 from April 2001.[24] User charges, therefore, seem likely to remain in place for the foreseeable future, though there may be changes to the complex range of exemptions.

Conclusion

It is clear that we lack reliable information about a number of the health care services paid for by individuals out-of-pocket and by other routes. Equally, though, the contours that we have identified suggest that the level of spending may be significant. It is clear from the evidence presented in this chapter that there is substantial health care activity outside the NHS, which is financed out-of-pocket rather than by conventional medical insurance. Indeed, the totality of the retail markets is larger than the private medical insurance market, and so deserves to be discussed alongside it.

The descriptive material assembled in this chapter and Chapter 2 show clearly that private health care financing and provision represent a very considerable proportion of total health care funding and service delivery in the UK, despite the dominant position of the NHS. Combining figures for the private supply and private funding of health care, including the provision of nursing home places (about £2 billion in 1996) and the supply of pharmaceuticals and medical equipment (about £3 billion in 1996), Laing[25] estimated that the total expenditure came to £14.5 billion (or 19.9 per cent) of total UK health care expenditure. This figure cannot readily be compared to the NHS budget of £40 billion, not least because some of the private financing is spent within the

NHS (e.g. in pay beds and as user charges). But it does suggest that the public–private balance is tilted more towards the private side of the equation than is generally realised. The scale of the non-NHS sector and its inter-relationships with the NHS confirms the view that health policy must be made increasingly with an eye on both sectors.

References

1   Wagstaff A, van Doorslaer E. Equity in the delivery of health care: some international comparisons. *J Health Economics* 1992; 11: 389–411.

2   Data supplied by the Proprietary Association of Great Britain. Figure is for calendar year 1997, and does not include medicines usually defined as complementary.

3   Barnett N, Denham M, Francis S-A. Over-the-counter medicines and the elderly. *Journal of the Royal College of Physicians* 2000; 34: 445–6.

4   Blenkinsopp A, Bradley C. Patients, society and the increase in self-medication. *BMJ* 1996; 312: 629–32.

5   House of Lords Science and Technology Committee. *Complementary and Alternative Medicine*. HL 123, Session 1999–2000. London: Stationery Office, 2000.

6   Wittenberg R. Economics of Long-Term Care Finance. In: *Royal Commission on Long-Term Care. With respect to old age*. Research Volume 1. Cm 4192–II/I. London: Stationery Office, 1999: 38.

7   National Audit Office. *Charitable Funds Associated with NHS Bodies*. HC 516, Parliamentary Session 1999–00. London: Stationery Office, 2000.

8   National Lottery Charities Board. *Annual Report 1999–2000*. London: National Lottery Charities Board, 2000: 9.

9   Department of Health. *Departmental Report 2000*. London: Stationery Office, 2000.

10 Proprietary Association of Great Britain (personal communication).

11 Health Committee. *The Regulation of Private and Other Independent Healthcare*. Volume I. London: Stationery Office, 1999.

12 Ibid.

13 Professions Allied to Medicine and Related Grades of Staff (PT'A') Council. *Staff Side Evidence 1998*. London: Chartered Society of Physiotherapy, 1998.

14 Thomas K, Fall M, Parry G, Nicholl J. *National Survey of Access to Complementary Health Care via General Practice*. Sheffield: University of Sheffield, Medical Care Research Unit, 1995.

15 Health Committee. *The Regulation of Private and Other Independent Healthcare*. Volume I. London: Stationery Office, 1999.

16 Luff D, Thomas K. *Models of Complementary Therapy Provision in Primary Care*. Sheffield: ScHARR, 1998.

17 Thomas K, Fall M, Parry G, Nicholl J. *National Survey of Access to Complementary Health Care via General Practice*. Sheffield: University of Sheffield, Medical Care Research Unit, 1995.

18 Laing and Buisson. *Health Cash Plans UK. Market sector report 2001*. London: Laing and Buisson, 2001: 1.

19 Lattimer M. *The Gift of Health*. London: Directory of Social Change, 1996.

20 National Audit Office. *Charitable Funds Associated with NHS Bodies*. HC 515, Session 1999–2000. London: Stationery Office, 2000: 1.

21 Department of Health. *Departmental Report 2000*. London: Stationery Office, 2000.

22 Federation of Ophthalmic and Dispensing Opticians. *Optics at a Glance*. London: FODO, 2000.

23 Government Statistical Service. *Optical Voucher Survey 1998*. London: NHS Executive, 1999.

24 Department of Health. *Prescription charge increase is lowest percentage increase for over 20 years*. Press Release 2001/0135, 16 March 2001.

25 Laing and Buisson. *Laing's Healthcare Market Review 1999–2000*. London: Laing and Buisson, 1999.

Chapter 4

Boundaries in health care: beyond the public–private divide

Introduction

In this chapter we explore public–private boundaries in more detail, focusing on the extent to which they are both blurred and shifting, with the picture becoming more complicated as the Labour Government seeks to create new public–private partnerships. The analysis shows that boundaries are becoming more permeable and that their location has shifted appreciably in the last 20 years. The primary, but not exclusive, effect has been to narrow the scope of the NHS in a mostly unplanned way as it has attempted to cope with increasing demands upon it. One solution to the perceived increasing gap between what the NHS can afford and the range of treatments available is to advocate an extended role for private finance and provision. A number of such approaches are discussed. Examples of people and resources that cross boundaries are used to illustrate the issues that policy-makers will need to address now that public and private health care are jointly on the Government's policy agenda. Whatever their intellectual appeal, they may be politically unattractive since they would require the Government to define in detail the range of health services which should be publicly financed and those which should be left to individuals to decide and access for themselves.

Nevertheless, this is not to say that nothing can be done to alter the current public–private boundaries and their regulation in the UK. As noted in earlier chapters, UK policy-makers have historically devoted relatively little time to health care issues outside the NHS, or to the implications of the existence of state-sponsored and private systems alongside one another. Now, the NHS Plan confirms that much greater attention will be paid to these issues in the future.[1] The historical lack of attention means that there are many problems in terms of equity of access and the protection of patients' interests that have yet to be tackled.

Blurred boundaries

The data presented in Chapter 2 focused attention on the different combinations of public and private financing and the provision of health care that currently exist in the UK. There are, however, a number of important dimensions that cannot easily be fitted into the four quadrants of Table 2.1 in Chapter 2, for example:

- some activity exhibits characteristics of both 'public' and 'private' working, such as private treatment provided in NHS pay beds
- when the same people work in both public and private settings, as in the case of hospital consultants and general dentists
- when the ways in which resources are used across the public and private sectors as a whole are not well-understood, as is presently the case with health cash plans.

At its simplest, a boundary is the place where a system meets its environment. For most of Chapter 2, the discussion was implicitly about formal boundaries, which could be defined in legal terms. We need to bear in mind, however, that boundaries are not always where we think they are. Moreover, there may not be universal agreement as to their nature or importance.

Burchardt and colleagues[2,3] recognised that although the four quadrant schema of Table 2.1 in Chapter 2 is useful, it fails to describe some important activities accurately. Therefore, they propose an additional dimension, in which the purchasing of services (i.e. the demand side of the system) is split into two parts, i.e. 'finance' and 'decision' (Figures 4.1 and 4.2). 'Finance' refers to the source of the resources and so may be public or private. 'Decision'-making may also be public or private, with the distinction being made between:

- a situation in which the choice is made by the consumer from a range of services that are (ideally) similar in price and quality (private decision)
- a situation where decisions are taken by a public body, or by agents acting on behalf of consumers (public decision).

Thus, private decisions include those made by individuals who purchase publicly provided services for which fees are charged. Private decisions would also occur if publicly financed vouchers enabled people to 'shop around' for other services (e.g. for child care), and do occur in the purchase of privately provided services, such as over-the-counter medicines.

Figure 4.1 Classification of public and private welfare activity

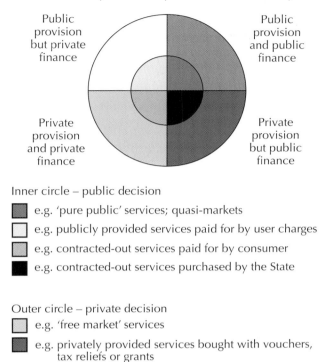

Public
provision
but private
finance

Public
provision
and public
finance

Private
provision
and private
finance

Private
provision
but public
finance

Inner circle – public decision

☐ e.g. 'pure public' services; quasi-markets
☐ e.g. publicly provided services paid for by user charges
☐ e.g. contracted-out services paid for by consumer
☐ e.g. contracted-out services purchased by the State

Outer circle – private decision

☐ e.g. 'free market' services
☐ e.g. privately provided services bought with vouchers,
     tax reliefs or grants
☐ e.g. publicly provided services bought with vouchers
☐ e.g. publicly provided services bought by individuals

Source: Burchardt T *et al. Private Welfare and Public Policy*, 1999: 10.

Figure 4.2 Expenditure on health

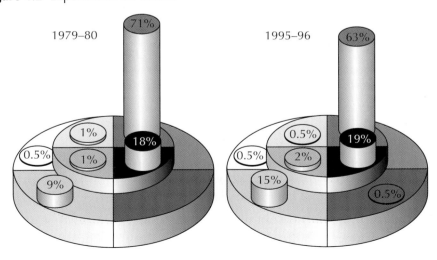

Source: Burchardt T *et al. Private Welfare and Public Policy*, 1999: 11.

Burchardt *et al.*[4] describe public–private boundaries in welfare financing and provision as 'fuzzy' when the additional dimension of 'decision' is taken into account, and state that the difference between the outer ring and inner circle in Figure 4.1 is a matter of degree. Figure 4.1 is therefore a practical device for clarifying the nature of complicated public–private relationships. It allows many different 'cross-boundary' flows to be placed on the same diagram, and highlights the many types of relationship that exist. To show how this blurring of boundaries manifests itself in health care, the examples of NHS pay beds, consultants, GPs, and individuals who use private health care will be discussed.

NHS pay beds

NHS pay beds were created as part of the settlement with the medical profession at the founding of the NHS. In order to get the hospital side of the NHS up and running, and in return for agreeing to work as salaried employees in NHS hospitals, consultants were allowed to practise privately alongside their NHS work. They were allowed to treat patients in private beds located within NHS hospitals, and to bill for the treatment provided. Today, about 100,000 patients (or 2.4 per cent of all inpatients) are treated in NHS pay beds each year.[5]

Pay-bed patients use NHS theatres and other facilities, which are charged for and included in pay-bed prices. Thus, pay beds are 'islands' of private practice within the NHS, relying on NHS facilities, but also providing a source of NHS income. They have periodically been highly contentious, with much discussion of their very existence within the NHS, and the fact that they enable private patients to buy earlier or more conveniently timed treatment, and additional amenities not available to NHS patients. There has been further argument as to whether NHS patients benefit from the presence of pay beds because of the income they generate or, conversely, whether the NHS suffers because the costs are not fully recognised and charged.

Pay beds are to be used in accordance with guidance published by the (then) Department of Health and Social Security in 1986 (*Health Services Management: Private Practice in Health Service Hospitals*), more commonly known as the 'Green Book'. The 'Green Book' states that pay beds should be managed to ensure they do not make financial losses (i.e. pay beds must not lead to unplanned subsidising of the private sector by the public sector). In practice, they have tended to make modest surpluses for NHS hospitals each year. The 'Green Book' also contains a statement of six principles which make it clear that pay-bed treatment should not compromise the equity objectives of the NHS:

- The provision of accommodation and services for private patients should not significantly prejudice non-paying patients.
- Subject to clinical considerations, earlier private consultation should not lead to earlier NHS admission or earlier access to NHS diagnostic procedures.
- Common waiting lists should be used for urgent and seriously ill patients, and for highly specialised diagnosis and treatment. The same clinical criteria should be used for categorising paying and non-paying patients.
- After admission, access by all patients to diagnostic and treatment facilities should be governed by clinical considerations.
- Standards of clinical care and services provided by the hospital should be the same for all patients. However, this does not affect the provision, on separate payment, of extra amenities.
- Single rooms should not be held vacant for potential private use longer than the usual time between NHS patient admissions.

The creation of NHS Trusts in the NHS and Community Care Act 1990 raised questions about the status of pay beds because NHS Trusts were given greater discretion in running them than the NHS had previously been allowed. The 'Green Book' was not withdrawn, but appears to have been shelved. Trusts were encouraged to raise some of their own funds and pay beds were viewed as a potential source of revenue. The period after 1991 saw many Trusts concentrate their pay beds, which had often been dispersed across many wards, into discrete pay-bed units. In a small number of cases, pay beds were sub-contracted to a private provider, further nuancing their already ambiguous status. However, these beds remained legally part of the NHS and should have remained subject to NHS rules. Allowing differences to grow up in waiting times creates incentives to use pay beds in preference to other NHS beds.

Notwithstanding the uncertainty over the effects of the 1990 Act, it seems reasonable to ask whether the 1986 'Green Book' guidance on not compromising treatment for NHS patients has been followed. The answer appears to be 'no'. Williams[6] analysed NHS Hospital Episode Statistics data for the period 1989–95 and found that median waiting times for all ordinary admissions had risen from 34 to 42 days, while for private patients the waiting time had fallen from 11 to 9 days. This broad pattern was true for a range of conditions, including some that are usually viewed as urgent such as breast excisions (*see* Table 4.1). The 'Green Book' requirement to maintain common waiting lists for non-elective patients was, as far as we could establish, not being met. This is hardly surprising given that the main point of paying for private treatment in the UK is to secure treatment more quickly than in the NHS.

Table 4.1 Median waiting times to elective admission for NHS pay beds and all NHS beds (inpatients and day cases), 1994–95*

Operation	OPCS4R Code	NHS Pay beds (days)	All NHS beds (days)
Operation on coronary artery	K40-51	13	76
Excision of breast	B27-28	7	15
Operation on inguinal hernia	T19-21	13	86
Prosthesis of lens	C75	17	175
All patients with surgical operation		10	46

*Adapted from Williams B. *Health Trends* 1997; 29: 21–5.

Contrary to appearances, Williams argues that the presence of pay beds may not be compromising NHS care, not least because the scale of the NHS dwarfs pay-bed provision. Strictly speaking, this view is correct, as no causal relationship has been demonstrated between the rates of pay-bed and normal NHS admissions. But it is clear that the criteria set out in the 'Green Book' are being violated, and that pay beds are a clear-cut example of a two-tier clinical service within the NHS hospital system, irrespective of whether or not pay-bed patients should be able to purchase additional amenities not available to NHS patients.

Pay beds embody many of the tensions inherent in current public–private relations. Even with the formal ending of the NHS internal market, they remain attractive to NHS hospitals because they provide income that can be used to treat more public patients as well as to keep consultants on site. They are also presumably attractive to consultants because they provide convenient access to private practice. While some insurance firms, including BUPA, do not cover pay beds, most do so. One attraction for insurers is that pay-bed units tend to offer lower prices than nearby free-standing private hospitals. Norwich Union – now part of CGNU – advertised an NHS pay bed-based product heavily in the London area in 1999, which was specifically tailored to the use of NHS pay beds in London teaching hospitals. The insurer was using the reputation of London teaching hospitals for high-quality care to promote a private medical insurance product, presumably with the support of the hospitals concerned, and guaranteeing its customers faster admission than NHS patients to non-pay beds in the same hospitals.

The equity theme of this book is echoed in the 'Green Book's' six principles. Pay beds are attractive to insurers and consultants, but evidence shows that there are violations and they do not guide current practice nearly as completely as they might. We recommend that the six 'Green Book' principles should be converted into performance standards. Indeed, some of the principles could be used to inform a wider debate about access to the NHS and the role of private health care. For example, the notion that time to admission should not be influenced by whether or not someone is paying for a service is a statement about horizontal equity. Even the more generally worded principles, such as that pay beds should not 'significantly prejudice' non-paying patients, raise questions about the extent of inequity generated by the remainder of the privately funded health sector that society is prepared to tolerate.

The NHS consultants' contract and private practice

If there is a single topic in this whole debate that has attracted comment from policy analysts in recent years, it is the freedom of consultants to maintain NHS and private practice in parallel. The majority of consultants in the UK have their main contract with the NHS, of which there are two main types:

- Consultants with full-time NHS contracts are permitted to earn up to 10 per cent of their NHS income on non-NHS work. By convention, their commitments are calculated in terms of notional half days (NHDs). Thus, full-time consultants work 11/11 of their time in the NHS.
- Consultants with maximum part-time contracts (10/11) or other fractional part-time contracts – the last often comprises consultants with academic posts – are free to earn such private income as they wish.

The NHS contract requires all consultants to fulfil their NHS commitments, and any non-NHS work should not compromise these commitments.

Neither contract specifies, however, what these requirements mean in practice. The contract is not tightly defined, being based on notions of trust between the State and doctors, and does not seek to prescribe work patterns in any detail. National guidelines state that:

a consultant on a whole-time or maximum part-time contract, between five and seven notional half days, depending on the specialty, should normally be allocated to fixed commitments.[7]

But 'fixed' commitments are not well defined, beyond the implication that they should be concerned with clinical work. Nor is the other type of commitment, termed 'flexible', and covering activities such as research and clinical audit. It is difficult, therefore, to be precise about what consultants need to do to fulfil their NHS commitments. In addition, it is not known how consultants actually fulfil their sessional commitments to the NHS.[8] In 1995, the Audit Commission reported that many NHS Trusts did not closely monitor the work of consultants, and felt that monitoring should be substantially improved.[9] Supporting this point, the Health Committee of the House of Commons published a report on the consultants' contract in the summer of 2000, in which it stated that:

Fixed sessions are vital because they give the most unambiguous statement of what work consultants do, and when ... there seemed to be no good reason for the wide variability in the number of fixed sessions specified. We agree [with the Audit Commission] that there should be a presumption in favour of consultants performing seven fixed sessions.[10]

There is evidence from self-reporting surveys[11] that many consultants work hard, and, for the vast majority, the total time they spend in the NHS more than reflects their contractual commitments. However, a minority may be under-serving the NHS. The Audit Commission[12] found evidence that NHS operating lists were sometimes postponed because a consultant was not available (and not away from work for illness or any other legitimate reason). It was also found that surgeons were not always supervising the training of the next generation, and sometimes undertaking very few NHS operations each week (*see below*). It is possible – though direct evidence was lacking – that consultants were unavailable to the NHS because they were undertaking private work.

There are about 27,000 consultants and specialists in the UK, 8000 of whom work only in the NHS and do no private work at all. Some consultants work entirely privately; it is difficult to estimate their numbers or the volume of work they undertake, but the Monopolies and Mergers Commission (MMC) estimated that in 1993 there were about 2500, the majority probably having retired from NHS practice. In terms of boundary management, the 17,000 who maintain a private practice alongside NHS work are of greater interest. An interview survey was undertaken in 1993 by the MMC of 556 consultants from a total of 612 approached. The results showed that, in a typical working week, 76 per cent undertook between 5 and 15 hours of private practice, with a total of between 40 and 80 hours spent in either NHS or private work[13] (see Table 4.2). In a typical week, 10 per cent of those interviewed worked for 15–19 hours, and 10 per cent for 20 or more hours, in private practice.

Table 4.2 Mean weekly hours spent by consultants on NHS and private practice, 1992

Consultants	NHS hours	Private practice hours	Total hours	Number of consultants in sample
Whole-time	53	6	59	58
Maximum part-time	51	11	62	404
Less than maximum part-time	45	16	61	70
Retired	2	38	40	29

Source: Monopolies and Mergers Commission. *Private Medical Services,* 1995: 52..

Income data is one source of information about the extent of private work. Figures 4.3 and 4.4 show the median incomes of full-time and maximum part-time consultants in 1993–94, derived from an Inland Revenue survey conducted for the Department of Health. The figures comprise salaried NHS income (Schedule E in Inland Revenue terms) and additional income (Schedule D). The data for full-time consultants show that many of them were earning more than the permitted 10 per cent over and above their NHS incomes, i.e. they were breaking the terms of their contracts. The data for maximum part-time consultants showed that they were undertaking an amount of work that almost doubled their NHS incomes, as they were allowed to do.

Consultants are able to increase their income by this extent because they charge far higher rates in private practice. The MMC estimated the mean hourly rates in 1992–93 for consultants in a number of specialties (see Figure 4.5). The lowest figure, £86 per hour for general medicine, was over three times higher than the estimated mean hourly rate of £25 per hour earned in the NHS by a consultant working on a maximum part-time contract.

It is reasonable, therefore, to ask whether consultants' private work affects their commitment to their NHS priorities. Data presented in Chapters 2 and 3

Figure 4.3 Full-time consultants

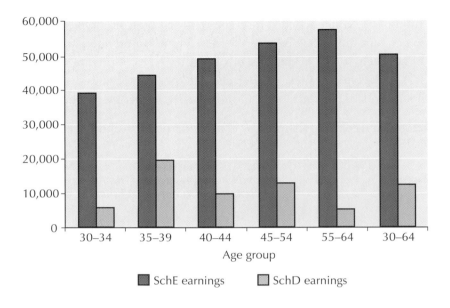

Figure 4.4 Maximum part-time consultants

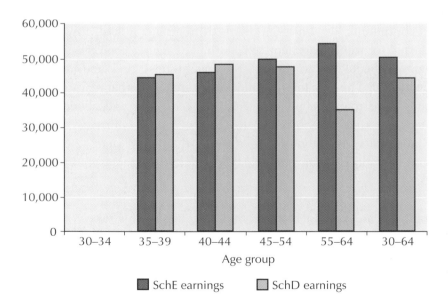

show that consultants' private activity is concentrated mainly in surgical specialties. The figures on private income and volume show that consultants who choose to do private work earn significant amounts from private practice,

Figure 4.5 Mean implied gross hourly rates earned from private practice and mean hours per week worked in private practice in certain specialties

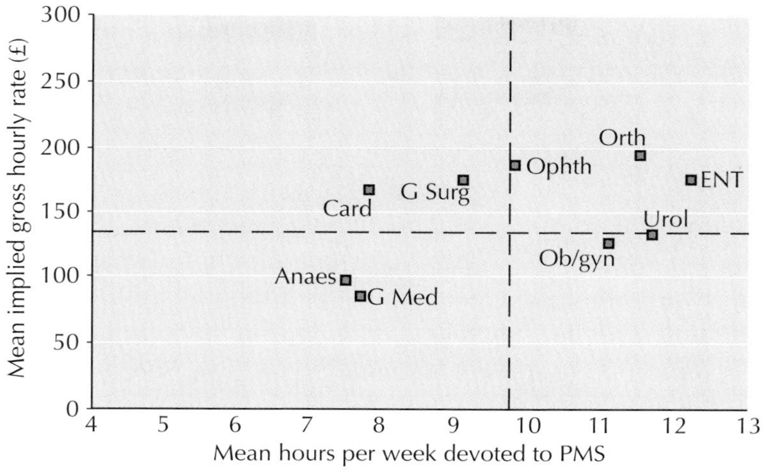

Source: Monopolies and Merger Commission. *Private Medical Services,* 1995: 54.

and that private practice is therefore very attractive to those who want it. The current NHS consultants' contract contains little if anything to place a check on the amount of this activity. Perhaps more fundamentally, there is a clash between a salaried service in the NHS, in which income is guaranteed, irrespective of the volume of work undertaken, while fee-for-service remuneration in the private sector means that income is directly related to the number of treatments undertaken. In such circumstances, it is inevitable that there will be financial incentives to give preference to private work, notwithstanding any professional ethics to the contrary.

However, it is difficult to show that private work *directly* influences consultants' NHS work. The most substantial work in this area has been done by Yates over a number of years. He concludes that a minority of consultants has been abusing the scope for private work, and that this has worked to the detriment of their NHS practice. Yates has used analyses of data on treatment rates and waiting lists to provide circumstantial evidence that consultants with extensive private practices tend to have longer NHS waiting lists than colleagues with less or no private work.[14,15] This might be expected given the strong financial incentives to practice privately. However, as Yates himself acknowledges, the data cannot demonstrate a causal relationship between the availability of private practice income and longer NHS waiting lists, and few surgeons have acceded to collection of relevant data. It seems likely that the causes of any such relationship are complex. For example, it is plausible that specialists who are sought after in the private sector are also in demand in the NHS and would have longer NHS lists as a consequence, irrespective of their level of commitment to the NHS.

More subtly, Yates looked at how much time surgeons were spending in operating theatres in the NHS. He found that it was possible for consultant surgeons to operate for three or even four sessions (or roughly 10 to 14 hours) each week in the NHS, but to spend an average of only six to eight hours per week operating. Indeed, some orthopaedic surgeons operated for only one to three hours per week in the NHS.[16] It is possible that surgeons work short sessions in order to work elsewhere.

On the basis of statistical analysis of Family Expenditure Survey data, Propper et al.[17] argue that the type of NHS consultant contract chosen by specialists is also an important determinant of the use of private health care:

> The effect of a rise in the number of senior doctors who opt for part-time employment in the NHS probably operates on both the NHS and the private sector. It depresses the quality of NHS care since the stock of senior doctors is fixed in the short term, and raises the quality of private care by increasing the supply of doctors to the private sector.[18]

Taking a more direct approach, Yates has also demonstrated that a small minority of consultants failed to devote 'substantially the whole of [their] time' to the NHS as the contract requires[19] and were therefore breaking the terms of their contracts. This evidence was derived from a controversial study of the work patterns of individual consultants, some of whom were tracked secretly by dispatch riders who followed them from site to site during their working hours.

The Government has now made it clear that it believes consultants work hard for the NHS, but also that their contracts need to be reviewed. The Government wants to ensure that their expensively acquired skills are used equitably and efficiently when they are working for the NHS, that there should be more rewards linked directly to their NHS work, and that they should be made more accountable for their NHS work than at present. It is less clear, however, how policies relating to private work by NHS consultants will develop.[20,21] The NHS Plan proposed that newly qualified consultants should not undertake private work, possibly for seven years.[22] Yet there are also local Concordats with private hospitals for the provision of elective surgery to NHS patients – presumably these operations will be undertaken by consultants who also have NHS contracts.

In February 2001, the Government published more detailed proposals, which in effect offered consultants a trade-off in relation to private practice. In return for the five- to seven-year delay in access to private work, newly qualified consultants were offered higher starting salaries (typically £60,000 per year, up from £50,000). They were also offered immediate access to a new clinical excellence award scheme, which would replace the current discretionary points and distinction awards schemes. For consultants in general, the Government offered a wider range of contractual arrangements, including more flexible contracts for older consultants, though it made it clear that all new contracts would require consultants to agree detailed job plans with their employers and undergo regular appraisals. The proposals have met with strong criticism from specialists' representatives and it is uncertain what final changes will emerge, and how any new arrangement will work in practice to affect consultants' relationships with the NHS and public–private relationships more broadly.[23]

General practitioners

General practice is another service long located at a public–private boundary, but one that is very different to the boundary straddled by consultants. Salter[24] has argued that GPs should also be viewed as being in the private sector rather than the NHS, on the basis of their independent contractor status and ownership of their own premises (see Chapter 2, Tables 2.3 and 2.4). This is consistent with the way in which general practice is defined by official bodies. For example, the National Accounts, published by the Office for National Statistics, treat GPs and dentists as 'unincorporated businesses', which are part of the 'personal sector'.[25] This is distinct from the public sector, which includes bodies undertaking activities financed and provided by the State. Figure 4.2 reflects this, showing that 19 per cent of health services were privately provided but publicly financed and decided in 1995–96,[26] with 18 per cent of the total provision being general medical services (GMS) provided by GPs.

Nevertheless, there is a difference between the legal status of GPs and public perceptions of their role within the NHS. Most GPs are still independent contractors to the NHS. However, it is interesting to note the recent growth in salaried GPs working on pilot sites for personal medical services, though this has been from a very low starting point.[27] They typically own their practice premises, so that their premises are not strictly speaking part of the NHS.

Yet GPs typically earn well over 95 per cent of their income from the NHS, and if we visit a GP as a patient, then it seems that they are part of the NHS. Indeed, to many people, GPs *are* the NHS.

The blurriness of this boundary is further emphasised by the incongruous fact that GPs are independent contractors, yet part of the NHS occupational pension scheme. This arrangement can also be traced back to 1946.

In spite of the apparent complexity of this situation, it is interesting to note that NHS general practice, unlike the position of many NHS specialists, raises few serious equity problems due to public–private relationships (GP fundholding raised separate inequity issues that no longer exist). Despite the fact that the NHS GMS contract governing the work of most GPs places only a very general responsibility on GPs to provide health care as and when required, it effectively prevents GPs charging patients on their lists for their main clinical services. GPs are able to earn private income, e.g. by charging for insurance medicals and for working as police surgeons, but charging is restricted to non-NHS services. As a result, there is little or no scope for 'double-cover' private GMS practice. Instead, only a very small number of people attend purely private GPs who have no links with the NHS. As a result of these contractual differences, the economics of private general practice are not attractive. As noted in Chapter 3, there have been periodic attempts by private entrepreneurs to increase the volume of private general practice, but at present it remains a niche service since it requires GPs to give up the public capitation income that they would have received for looking after the same patients in the NHS. The result is that almost all UK citizens believe that their main contact with the NHS is with their NHS-financed GP. The Government is currently in negotiation with GPs over a new contract, so that the relative attractiveness of NHS and private practice might change in the future.

Patients who use private health care

Users of private health care in the UK represent another source of boundary blurring and raise boundary management issues, since almost all of them are also users of the NHS, many on a regular basis. The number of studies of individuals and families who use private health care is small, but they help explain why people use the private sector given the availability of a NHS. Calnan *et al.*[28] interviewed people who had private health insurance and found that there were a number of reasons why people had private insurance. One was that people were simply given it as a 'job perk'; its availability meant it was used because of the perceived advantages it conferred over the NHS in access and convenience. It was also purchased as a response to the perceived risk of deteriorating health status (though note the observation in Chapter 3 that pre-existing conditions are generally excluded from UK private medical insurance cover). From the viewpoint of this book, the most interesting finding concerned attitudes towards a mixed economy of hospital care:

> *Those of our respondents who purchased private health insurance … did not do so because of a commitment to the market and did not support the NHS because of a lack of choice. They decided to subscribe on pragmatic grounds, because of the lack of waiting and the perceived level of comfort offered by the private sector … Our respondents were pro-NHS in principle but took out private health insurance for practical reasons, while resenting the fact that they had to pay twice and wishing that they could get the service they wanted from the NHS.*[29]

Thus, people who take out their own private medical insurance seem to support both NHS and private care, though they may support the NHS less strongly than those who do not have it. Calnan *et al.* suggest this is because they consume both types of health care, and might consume less private care if they judged that the NHS could provide what they wanted when they wanted it. This conclusion echoes the findings of Burchardt *et al.*,[30] who studied changes in the pattern of use of public and private services in education, housing and personal care in the 1980s and 1990s. They found that many of the people who used private provision also reported recent use of public services. Their pattern of use appeared to be flexible and pragmatic.

Turning to an even less well-researched area, we realised during the course of the research for this book that people who have access to private health care, through insurance or direct payment, can move advantageously between private treatment and the NHS, e.g. by seeing a consultant rapidly as a private outpatient, thereby receiving an earlier referral for NHS inpatient treatment. (Many insurance policies cover outpatient treatment and so make this possible, though they do not overtly encourage it.) Figures are not available on the extent to which this occurs, but there are anecdotal accounts of people moving seamlessly between NHS and private treatment for specialist services, where some services are available only in the NHS. Accessing NHS radiotherapy as part of a private course of cancer treatment is one example of this type of movement. In such cases, patients who are otherwise 'private' make use of the NHS for an essential part of their treatment. This enables the individual to gain maximum advantage from both sectors and enables the insurer to continue to provide selective cover, knowing that the NHS will deal with the high-cost or complex part of the treatment. For these patients, the NHS–private boundary may be all but invisible at times, but the impact on those who do not have access to private options may be appreciably less positive. This is an inevitable consequence of a situation in which people have access to two health care systems, one of which provides selective, incomplete cover and the other attempts to provide complete, but accordingly less well-defined cover.

Permeable boundaries

The overall picture is of selectively permeable boundaries between the NHS and the private health care sector. At some points, and for some people, including clinicians (with the inclination and in the right specialty) and patients (with private medical insurance or the ability to pay out-of-pocket), the boundary is easily crossed. At other points, such as general practice, it is not so easily permeable, and people stay either within the NHS or outside it. Patients who do not have the ability to pay depend on the NHS. Expensive services such as radiotherapy are typically available only in the NHS.

The example of general practice makes the point that public–private boundaries in themselves need not be a problem either for equity or consumer protection. The right contractual forms can lead to equitable arrangements with reasonable consumer protections built into them. This contrasts with the position of many NHS consultants with appreciable private practices. In their case, clinical work in the two sectors is inescapably inter-related, posing problems for any government committed to improving equity of access to services through the NHS. For example, the Labour Government's proposals to limit specialists' access to private work is likely to reduce the use of private hospital services and the take-up of private medical insurance (*see above*).

Shifting boundaries

The public–private boundary has also shifted significantly in some places in recent years. As a result, what is practically included in and excluded from the NHS has changed over time.[31] In this section, we briefly review trends in services where particularly notable recent shifts have taken place, to furnish more clues about why boundaries are located in particular places.

Long-term care of older people

Perhaps the most important shift of services out of the NHS came in the long-term care of older people in the 1980s. A number of apparently disparate policies came together, which had the effect of moving substantial elements of nursing care from the fully funded NHS to the private and voluntary nursing and residential care sector, in which access to care was either via means-testing or paid for entirely out-of-pocket. In the early 1980s, the Government decided that it was no longer appropriate to provide long-stay care for older people in hospital settings, and a programme of closing wards and whole hospitals was initiated, with the aim of providing more modern NHS facilities. The role of the district general hospital was increasingly seen as providing short-term care for acute conditions. Hospitals were also under increasing pressure to improve their 'productivity', which could be demonstrated by reducing lengths of stay and increasing patient throughput. Both goals were incompatible with providing long-term care.

In parallel with these NHS developments, local authorities had been responding to increasing demand for residential places since the 1970s by paying for a growing number of older people to be accommodated in private or voluntary residential and nursing homes. In the early 1980s, changes were made in social security rules that made it possible for people to receive board and lodging allowances from the State while resident in private and voluntary homes.[32] As Parker notes:

> One could hardly have devised a more effective combination of circumstances for encouraging a rapid development of the private sector of residential care for the elderly. It is tempting to conclude, therefore, that it all happened by design and in line with the Government's general view about the virtues of non-statutory forms of care. Such a conclusion is probably wrong. There seems little evidence that these changes were intended to accelerate private sector growth – or at least not on any substantial scale.[33]

One important result of the changes was that nursing care came to be provided to many thousands of older people in private and voluntary sector settings, whereas previously the generally frailer proportion of these people would have been receiving free nursing care and accommodation in NHS long-stay facilities. People found themselves paying for nursing care as part of the costs of their institutional care, even though they would have received it free through the NHS under previous arrangements (e.g. as on a long-stay ward in a district hospital).

Over time, this shift of long-term nursing care from the NHS, where it was free at the point of use, to the means-tested social care sector, came under ever-increasing fire.[34] The eventual result was the appointment of a Royal Commission on Long-Term Care, which reported in 1999 and recommended that all personal care – including nursing care but going beyond it – should be free.[35] This would have extended the scope of the State's commitment to financing long-term care considerably beyond the extent of its pre-1980s commitment, with major public spending implications. The Government published its broad response as part of the NHS Plan.[36] It accepted most of the Royal Commission's recommendations, and agreed that nursing care should be free wherever it was delivered. However, it did not accept that all 'personal care' should be free, and chose instead to fund only care provided by registered nurses. The NHS boundary has therefore moved outwards again, albeit relatively modestly.

Mental health services

Moving to other services, one of the most striking shifts in provision, but not funding, in the last decade has occurred in acute psychiatric care. The Health Committee of the House of Commons noted in 1999 that:

> *The number of premises and beds within the independent mental health sector has increased significantly over the last decade. The Royal College of Psychiatrists estimates that the sector now provides approximately 20 per cent of all acute psychiatric care, 81 per cent of all brain injury services, 30 per cent of medium secure care, 44 per cent of residential care for people with learning difficulties and 67 per cent of beds for non-acute mental health care in registered mental nursing homes and residential homes.*[37]

This contribution to NHS services from the non-governmental sector is a recent phenomenon. The precise origins of the shift are not well documented, although part of the reason for it appears to be related to the introduction of the NHS internal market in 1991. Some health authorities (particularly in metropolitan areas) found that they did not have adequate facilities for these groups. Yet, neither did they have easy access to capital to increase their mental health facilities within the NHS. The emphasis was on re-provision of former hospital facilities in community settings, but this required a source of investment capital that was not forthcoming. In response to this difficulty, some health authorities used the extra-contractual referral mechanism to place interim contracts with private providers. However, once in place, these contractual relationships were sustained, resulting in a new pattern of publicly funded non-NHS provision.

General dental services

There are yet more examples of substantial shifts from state to private provision. Table 2.2 in Chapter 2 shows that 20 per cent of general dentistry is now privately financed and provided, with a further 23 per cent privately financed and publicly supplied. The 23 per cent figure largely reflects the rising proportion of total costs met from co-payments made by NHS patients for general dentistry since 1951. The 20 per cent figure for privately financed and provided dentistry is of more recent origin. In 1992–93, 5 per cent of treatments were financed and provided privately,[38] yet the proportion had risen up to 20 per cent by 1996–97.

The main reason for the change appears to have been a falling out between the dental profession and the Conservative Government of the time over the terms of a new NHS dental contract. Increases in the number of dentists in the late 1980s had led to a substantial increase in activity and expenditure that the Government had responded to by imposing cash limits on the NHS general dental budget for the first time, from 1990, as they sought to rein-in expenditure. It also sought to introduce a new dental contract setting out revised terms of service for dentists. The changes included revised fee scales in order to encourage preventive rather than restorative work.

Thus, the Government was attempting to both 'claw back' what it perceived as over-expenditure, and at the same time negotiate new terms and conditions. The result was, however, that dentists were aggrieved at what they saw as shabby treatment, and unattractive new rates of remuneration.[39] Dentists in more affluent areas, where patients were willing and able to pay, stopped offering NHS services to adults (though they generally maintained NHS services for children).

The result today is a mixed economy of both financing and provision in dentistry, where previously there had been a much stronger emphasis on NHS provision, albeit with substantial patient co-payments. The most important result has been that some people now find it difficult to access an NHS dentist, particularly in more affluent areas where dentists are only prepared to offer private services to adults. For adults, dental health care services have largely slipped out of the NHS in many parts of the country, almost by accident, leading to serious access problems for some low-income people.[40]

The Labour Government recognised that there were problems of access to dentistry, and published a dental strategy in Autumn 2000.[41] The strategy estimated that up to 2 million people were having difficulty accessing NHS dental treatment, though the basis of this estimate was not clear. It promised – as the Prime Minister had done in late 1999 – that everyone who wanted it would be able to have NHS dental treatment by September 2001. There were proposals that might contribute to better access, such as new walk-in dental treatment centres. However, these centres will only treat about 50,000 patients each year (i.e. 50 centres treating about 10,000 patients each). The strategy does little to address the core problem, which is the lack of dentists to meet the demand for NHS treatment.

From our point of view, the key point is that the Government has had an opportunity to remedy an access problem. It has made some moves in the right direction – the walk-in centres ought to help – but has neither tackled the underlying problems of capacity and levels of financing in the NHS system nor the resulting balance of public and private financing and provision. The dental strategy is interesting too, because it reveals the Government as making policy for the NHS, rather than for the dental service as a whole.

Ophthalmic services

A final example of shifting boundaries can be found in general ophthalmic services. A Conservative government ended free NHS eyesight tests for the whole population in 1989. Children and some classes of adults (e.g. people on certain qualifying benefits) continued to have free tests paid for by the NHS. By the late 1990s, almost 50 per cent of eyesight tests were financed and provided privately. As in the case of the nursing component of long-term care, the boundaries are now shifting back. The Labour Government restored free eyesight tests for people aged 60 years and over in April 1999. The result was a 34 per cent increase in NHS tests in the following 12 months, the bulk of which were performed on older people.[42] As in the case of dentistry, the Government has recognised a problem and acted, but has not gone as far as it might have done by restoring the pre-1989 arrangements.

Assessing and learning from boundary blurring and boundary changes

It was noted in earlier chapters that much of the blurring of boundaries can be traced back to the compromises underlying the 1946 NHS Act. The examples of boundary shifts discussed above also point to a more recent history of substantial increases in the proportion of private provision and finance of some services. However, the reasons for the shifts were not the same in each case. In some cases, change was planned, as with the withdrawal of free eyesight tests on grounds of low priority and their subsequent partial re-introduction. By contrast, the increase in both privately provided and funded nursing home care and in privately provided acute psychiatric services appears to have been largely unplanned, although it may not have been unwelcome to the Conservative governments of the day. Similarly, the changes in dentistry appear not to have been planned. However, again, there is more than a hint that general dental services for adults are regarded by different governments as a low priority for support, justifiably or not.

The result of the shifts described above is that more services are mixed in terms of both financing and provision than 20 years ago. As a result, there are now three main models of health care in the UK system (leaving aside the retail markets discussed in Chapter 3). The models are:

- Services that are financed and provided mainly by the NHS
- Services financed mainly by the NHS, but with mixed public and private provision. These include the psychiatric services discussed earlier, and some elective surgery
- Mixed economies of financing and provision, as in general dentistry and long-term care.

The 1946 Settlement, while still in place, has been amended over time. Eighty-four per cent of services are still financed and provided by the NHS, so that patients are still mainly treated free at the point of delivery, but there is a greater role for private provision than before. Seen in this light, the Labour Government's NHS Plan simply formalises a set of relationships that have been emerging over recent years by explicitly recognising in policy terms the contribution of private provision to the treatment of NHS patients.

One consequence of the unplanned nature of many changes is the absence of conscious policy decisions about which services should be financed or provided by the NHS, and which by the private sector. There are many service arrangements that have developed to suit local or particular circumstances. As a result, there is no single overall rationale for the current patterns of public and private sector interdependence. An alternative would be to develop a more consistent pattern of services and regulation.

New and Le Grand[43,44] argue that these questions can sometimes be resolved through analysis and judgement, according to cost-effectiveness and other criteria. For example, one set of criteria might be that if an intervention has to be undertaken by a health professional and can be shown to be cost-effective, it should be funded by the NHS on grounds of efficiency and patient protection. They go on to note, however, that health care systems have not generally been built from first principles, but have simply evolved over time. As a result, practical policy-makers have to work with seemingly anomalous boundaries, which cannot easily be undone.

On the other hand, the accumulation of past decisions is not necessarily arbitrary, but reflects values that may not have been clearly articulated at any stage. Conscious decisions may not have been taken about the position of some services, but there may be relatively little pressure to shift them from their current position. As an example, New and Le Grand[45] suggest that general dentistry is a service that could be provided outside the NHS, as it is in other countries. Patients are relatively knowledgeable about their own oral health and need for treatment, and that dentistry has therefore some of the characteristics of a service that could be offered in a retail market. In addition, modern dentistry has a significant cosmetic component such that the State should not be required to finance it. They argue that such considerations may explain why general dentistry lies on the fringes of the NHS and why the reduction in the public proportion of financing of dental care has been met with relatively little demur. While these are tidy arguments, they are highly contestable. Patients are generally poorly informed about the precise nature of their needs for dental care as for other health services, and the dividing line between therapeutic and cosmetic treatment is by no means clear-cut. Real-life attempts – as in the debate about core health services in New Zealand – to define explicitly the boundaries between publicly and privately financed care have shown how difficult this can be, though as a matter of logic there must be *de facto* limits to what the NHS can provide.

Alternative solutions to the public–private balance

Despite the difficulty in practice of determining the boundary between public and privately funded provision, the belief that there is an inevitable widening 'gap' between what the NHS can provide and the demands placed upon it[46] provides the starting point for those who argue for a very different set of relationships between public and private sectors in the UK. For example, the increasing numbers of high-cost drugs, e.g. beta-interferon, Viagra, and so on, have led to contentious rationing decisions. These examples demonstrate, so the argument continues, that a publicly funded system, particularly one funded mainly from general taxation, cannot provide the level and standard of health care that an increasingly affluent, aged and sophisticated population wants (though there is no way to determine to everyone's satisfaction which level of spending is 'correct').

This account of the current situation is significantly true. After all, rationing does occur. Both Labour and Conservative governments have vowed to keep taxes and public spending under close control. The proportion of total spending on health services that is private has risen, albeit gradually in the last 20 years. This has encouraged some people to suspect that a government might at some point argue that private finance is the only way of increasing health care funding – the Private Finance Initiative is cited as an example here.

It is argued by those who would wish to alter the boundary between the public and private sectors radically, that the main difference between the UK and other comparable countries lies not in the level of public funding of its health care, but in the lower level of private funding that is constrained by the dominance of the NHS and its unfulfilled pretensions towards providing full cover to the whole population. At the same time, it is argued that substantial increases in public spending are not an option if the UK is to remain internationally, economically competitive, as well as being political suicide for any government. However, since individuals are on average better off, they should in principle be able to pay for more of their own health care. If better-off people are able to spend more of their money on health care outside the NHS, then inevitably the private sector will, and should, grow to meet the unmet demand in the public sector.

A range of 'solutions' to this long-term NHS funding 'crisis' has been offered, mostly involving some form of publicly financed 'core' of services available to all, with scope for the better-off to purchase a higher level of private cover for a wider range of services, thereby increasing the total amount spent on health care in the UK. Most alternatives to the current arrangements are based on an explicit rejection of the idea that the NHS can, or should, attempt to provide comprehensive health services for all, together with a very different role for private insurance.

One of the most sophisticated schemes has been proposed by Hoffmeyer and McCarthy[47] in a model that would replace the NHS. The model is based on both demand- and supply-side competition between both purchasers and providers of care. It proposes a form of social insurance, with sufficient insurance companies involved in the market to create competition for enrolment of citizens. Providers would compete for the business of insurance agency purchasers. Insurance premiums would reflect individuals' incomes and health risks (i.e. a hybrid of usual social insurance and conventional private medical insurance). There would be a prohibition on insurers excluding whole groups of patients or insisting on unreasonable terms to avoid risk. There would also be a central fund to equalise imbalances in income and risk-related contributions between insurance agencies (i.e. to share the costs of high-risk groups). These arrangements, it is argued, would be organised to provide a guaranteed basic package of health care for all, which all insurers have to offer. There should also be a safety net for individuals unable to cope or to find insurance.

This approach has something in common with the range of different forms of insurance in the UK before the NHS, but most particularly with elements of the current system in the Netherlands (*see* Chapter 6). The central ideas are enabling patients to choose between different packages of care and insurers, while being guaranteed access to a societally agreed basic package of care, and for better-off patients to be able to insure themselves for a higher level of care. This approach would increase the level of health care funding beyond the levels permitted by successive parsimonious governments. Behind the scenes, the Government would attempt to ensure that each insurer had roughly equal funds in relation to the requirements of its members.

Elements of this model can be found in proposals from other bodies, including the World Health Organisation.[48] The WHO advances what it calls a 'third-way' solution in health care, which is essentially a social insurance-based model with elements of competition between both purchasers and providers, and greater use of public–private partnerships. It is also echoed in a report from the Institute of Directors in the UK.[49] The Institute proposes an NHS 'passport' to basic services, with use of private medical insurance for 'top-up' payments for services provided over and above NHS core services.

There are further alternatives that proceed from different arguments. Bosanquet[50] identifies what he terms an 'effectiveness gap', manifested in the difference between what is possible and what is achieved. As examples, he cites access to services and service quality in the NHS for major illnesses, such as cancer and heart disease. He also argues that the NHS is poor at innovation compared to the private sector. Foreshadowing some of the Government's proposals in the NHS Plan, Bosanquet argues that there should be a range of public–private partnerships in the delivery of services, such that the strengths of public provision are retained while the private sector is used to innovate and provide competition in selected areas.

Irrespective of the intellectual merits of these schemes, governments in the UK have been reluctant to envisage a wholesale change to either the financing of care or the definition of the services to which public funding is meant to provide access. Part of their reluctance may spring from the difficulty of defining what would be a reasonable range and level of services to which all should be entitled ('core' services). Part may spring from a reluctance to depart from the ideal of the NHS providing equitably for everybody's needs, even though this is highly unlikely to be attainable. Hoffmeyer and McCarthy's model, for instance, requires explicit recognition in public policy that better-off people are likely to wish to purchase cover for a wider range of services than the public scheme can offer. It would not be straightforward to determine when private insurance was being used to purchase access to services *not* covered by the public scheme and when it was buying preferential access to services that *were* covered by the public scheme. Whether their model would be more or less equitable than the current public–private mix is not known. However, the resultant inequity would be explicit, since the State would be required to ensure the availability of defined 'core' services, whereas current arrangements in the UK, as we have seen in this chapter, have simply arisen *ad hoc* over time, leading to access anomalies between services.

Assessing the current public–private boundaries

It is our view that ambitious plans for an entirely different UK health system are not currently acceptable politically. Rather, the task is to determine whether the detail of the current complex balance of public and private funding and provision leads to a system that lives up to the two main principles of equity and consumer protection which guide the analysis in this book. Some of the services discussed in this chapter fall short of the equity benchmarks of Chapter 1. For example, the principle of universal access to services has been eroded in dentistry, where those people who are exempted from all payment towards their NHS treatment frequently cannot find an NHS dentist. The Government has recognised this problem and said that it will improve access, though it remains to be seen whether it will succeed.

The arrangements for long-term nursing care have clearly increasingly violated the principle of equitable access over the last 20 years. The Government is now restoring free nursing care to everyone who needs it,[51] and this involves defining nursing care for the first time. Nursing care will then satisfy the equity criterion in future, although older people will still be means-tested regarding their access to subsidy for the remainder of their personal care costs.

The other principle of consumer protection set out in Chapter 1 can also be a useful guide to assessing current public–private boundaries. Currently, some of the most vulnerable people in society are treated and cared for in private settings. This need not be a problem in itself if the State ensures that regulations protect their interests. The extent to which patient interests are fully protected and steps to improve current arrangements are discussed in Chapter 7.

The Government's position on public–private boundaries

The current government's response to the historical disposition of public and private financing and provision in the UK, as shown in the NHS Plan, is to retain and strengthen the NHS while being more explicit in its management of the relations between the public and private spheres of health care than any of its recent predecessors. Thus, its actions are more likely to conform to the two principles of equity of access for equal need and consumer protection than its recent predecessors.

The Government appears to have been favourably impressed by arguments setting out the advantages of a universal system that have been well described by many people down the years, from Aneurin Bevan onwards. The NHS offers good value for the money we spend on it, and the UK emerges favourably from international comparisons of equity and efficiency.[52] The NHS is a low-cost, efficient and reasonably equitable system. The NHS continues to attract high levels of public support: seventy-seven per cent of the population still supports the principle of a universal health service (though this does not necessarily mean that they oppose people having the choice of paying extra for private health care).[53] It may be hard to believe when you are on a long NHS waiting list, but citizens are relatively satisfied with the NHS compared with citizens of other countries, though the NHS is not the 'world leader' on this measure.[54]

The Labour Government has explicitly committed itself to supporting the NHS, the NHS Plan and the 2000 Budget.[55] It has accepted the argument that we can continue to fund health care without any great difficulty if we choose to do so, and has acted on it. This aspect of its plans, focusing on improving the NHS while rejecting a wider role for private insurance, represents continuity with the past, despite the fact that the rate of increase of NHS spending planned is unprecedented.

The novelty in the Government's plans is reflected in its tackling of two issues on the boundaries of the NHS: public–private partnerships and protocols, principally to govern access to private sector services for NHS patients; and the regulation of NHS consultants' access to private practice in parallel with their NHS work. The first signs of a major policy change came in a speech given by Alan Milburn in December 1999, soon after he became Secretary of State for Health.[56] The direction of change was confirmed by Prime Minster Tony Blair on BBC's *Newsnight* in February 2000, when he indicated that he had no ideological objection to the use of private providers by the NHS.

The NHS Plan, and a number of statements made by the Prime Minister and other ministers during 2001, confirms that there are now policies that extend beyond the NHS into private health care. On the financing side, the Government is hostile to the use of private medical insurance, and devoted an entire chapter of the Plan to arguing that it is both inefficient and inequitable.[57] This is hardly a surprising conclusion for a Labour government, but it is revealing that ministers wished to include such direct comment on a key plank in the 'double-cover' private market. On the other hand, the Government has stopped short of limiting its use directly. Indeed, there are no proposals for any policy initiatives with respect to the regulation of the private medical insurance market for the sake of consumer protection or equity. Instead, the Government is pursuing the more conventional line of improvements in NHS performance, particularly by aiming for shorter waiting times for treatment. Implicitly, the Government envisages that this will reduce the demand for private hospital care, and hence insurance, thereby indirectly making overall access to health care more equitable. The difference on the financing side compared with its predecessors is that it has a great deal of extra money to spend on improving the NHS and therefore of reducing the attractiveness of privately financed alternatives.

On the delivery side, there is the Concordat between the NHS and private providers of care, covering elective surgery, transfers from private hospitals to

NHS intensive care units, and intermediate care. These are in addition to the Private Finance Initiative, which enables the NHS to lease facilities built and owned by private developers on a long-term basis. Thus, the role of publicly financed, privately provided services is to be included in mainstream policy-making, along with a recognition of the reliance of the private sector on the NHS in the case of intensive care. The Plan is not detailed, and there remains room for discussion and debate about the nature of the Concordat. Ministerial statements during and after the 2001 General Election did not provide any further clarification. However, further blurring of the public–private distinction on the provision side can be expected.

In theory, the Government could have stopped at this point with the Concordat. In this case, the Plan would amount to little more than policies and practices already found in the NHS being formalised at the national level. After all, local NHS organisations already enter into pragmatic public–private partnerships. Indeed, if the NHS continues to face high private sector prices for elective surgery, then it may not extend its purchasing of private services much beyond its present level of about 85,000 procedures each year.[58] Private sector interest in developing intermediate care would, similarly, depend on commercial judgements about the benefits of entering the market at prices largely determined by the NHS.

However, the Government is also concerned to mitigate what it sees as the worst of the perverse incentives created by the fudge on which the NHS hospital sector was established, and wants to reduce *directly* the amount of private service delivery in order to improve equity of access to services. It proposes, albeit not as its last word on the subject, that consultants should not be able to practise outside the NHS for the first five or seven years after qualifying as a consultant, which would tend to reduce the supply of private treatment. This bold proposal contrasts with the Concordat, which suggests that the Government sees a continuing role for the private hospital sector, quite possibly as part of an overtly mixed economy of provision, enabling the NHS to gain access to spare capacity when it needs it.

Reducing the size of the privately financed sector by direct action to alter the NHS consultants' contract will be a far more difficult path to tread. At present, the pattern of private elective surgery, which accounts for most of NHS consultants' private practice, is to a significant extent controlled by surgeons. The Concordat for elective surgery risks simply cementing existing working practices in place. If the Government wishes to change working practices, in order to make overall access to health services more equitable, and in pursuit of its modernisation agenda, it will have to take greater control of surgeons' working practices. The Government recognises this, and presumably also appreciates the incendiary nature of the debate that has been stirred up by attempts to limit private practice. There may be legal challenges to such restrictions. Some consultants may leave the NHS and work exclusively in the private sector. Others may threaten to do so. Still others may 'work to rule' in order to demonstrate that they already work more than their contracted hours and have, therefore, earned the right to do as much private work as they see fit. Representative bodies are likely to argue that new NHS specialists will have to be paid considerably more by the NHS if their right to private practice is curtailed, a point which will be complicated by the fact that the scope for private practice varies markedly among different specialties.

The proposal that newly qualified consultants should not be allowed to practise privately for seven years is a crude one. One interpretation is that it is simply a means of signalling to the consultants that the Government means business. Another interpretation is that the Government knows that it will have to compromise in the difficult negotiations which lie ahead with the consultants and is therefore leaving itself plenty of room to reach a reasonable accommodation between public and private interests. In the eyes of prospective NHS consultant surgeons and anaesthetists who want private practice, most solutions would appear preferable to a blanket seven-year ban!

Direct regulation via the contract is not the Government's only route to altering consultants' behaviour. The Concordat can also be used to subject private hospitals and consultants to standards contained in National Service Frameworks and other NHS policy instruments. These could be used to constrain the working practices of consultants. The Plan notes that there will need to be better information exchange between the NHS and private sectors. Therefore, the Concordat might be used to provide the NHS with much better information about consultants' working practices. Another avenue for the NHS might be to negotiate access to private treatments directly with specialists of its choosing, selecting only those whom it judged to be working equitably and efficiently in the NHS and honouring their NHS commitments.

Creating a closer relationship between the NHS and private providers will also force a review of the regulation of provision. The Care Standards Act 2000[59] (see Chapter 7) still treats NHS and private providers differently. There are important anomalies in the current arrangements. For example, a private hospital with a contract to treat NHS patients will be regulated as a private establishment by the National Care Standards Commission. Yet patients will presumably, as at present, have access to NHS complaints mechanisms should any problem arise. The issue of integrating the regulation of public and private provider organisations in order to ensure consumer protection is covered in Chapter 7.

Towards a more sophisticated debate

The Government appears to have decided that the political fudges agreed at the time of the creation of the NHS are no longer sustainable. They need to be replaced with more transparent contracts between the State and the professions, and new agreements between the State and private providers, which together will allow the Government to honour a new social contract with patients – to provide a service that is fairer, more accessible and more sensitive to their needs. The Plan does not provide all the detail required to tell whether or not it will be successful in improving public–private boundaries in UK health care. Nevertheless, it establishes the basis for a more explicit discussion about the proper role of private health care than at any time in the recent past.

The transition from one set of long-standing relationships to another one may not be smooth. Private firms may perceive that there are opportunities to secure new sources of funding for their services and market themselves more aggressively than ever. If NHS managers sense that it is appropriate to agree contracts for radiology services, or some day-case procedures, then new markets could be created for privately provided services. Consultants are likely to resist changes to their NHS contracts designed to limit the extent of their private practices.

This makes it especially important for the Government to be clear about the principles it is using to direct its health services policies. We propose that equity of access should, as the NHS Plan 2000 implies, be a major focus of policy-making. The Plan makes strong statements about the inequitable effects of private medical insurance on provision – though it contains no new proposals for action – and the same arguments should be followed through by acting directly on access to services in the NHS. To do so, the Government will be faced with two challenges, both already alluded to. One is conceptual. Decisions would have to be made about services that currently sit astride the public–private health care boundary. Should they be publicly financed and provided, or publicly financed with mixed provision, mixed in terms of both financing and provision, or even solely privately financed and provided?

Noting New and Le Grand's argument that it is important to be clear about the values used in these areas, one way of making them explicit is to decide on the nature and extent of equity desired according to the benchmarks set out in Chapter 1. The solution for any one service may be different from others. It might be justifiable, for example, to decide that nursing care really must be free to all wherever it is provided, but that some dental treatments are primarily cosmetic and should be outside the NHS system (though it may still be desirable to regulate their provision).

The Government might also decide, for example, that it is justifiable in the name of equity to ensure that patients in NHS pay beds waited the same time for their treatment as other NHS patients.

The principle of the quality of consumer protection can also be used to guide thinking. As matters stand, the Government has indicated a move away from the previous *laissez-faire* policy towards active protection of consumer interests. It is not yet clear how far new regulations to be introduced under the Care Standards Act 2000[60] will actually succeed in this aim. It is possible, though, to imagine assessing any new set of regulations in terms of the protection they afford to patients in different settings. Sometimes it will be appropriate to allow people to determine their own need for treatment, and focus on making sure the service is safe and of good quality. At other times it will be necessary to regulate to protect consumers, because they will be exposed to financial or clinical risks that they themselves are poorly placed to assess.

Even if the problems noted here are successfully addressed, the new system will still contain important elements from the past. For example, it is almost unthinkable that any government will ban all 'double-cover' private medical insurance, except as part of a move to an entirely different type of health system, such as the Canadian one, in which private insurance is only permitted for services not covered by the public scheme. Thus, private insurance will still be available for services already covered by the NHS, ensuring an alternative route to health care that the Government can do nothing to make more equitable. In turn, NHS consultants might find their access to private practice more limited than at present, but they will still seek to protect their current control over public–private boundaries. The Concordat and other proposals in the NHS Plan will not therefore be a panacea because they will not deal with the private sector in its entirety (e.g. there is no discussion of public policy vis-à-vis private medical insurance). However, the NHS Plan does show that equity and consumer protection issues are beginning to be addressed by the Government across the boundaries between public and private sectors in a new way.

The next two chapters show how other countries with very different patterns of public and private financing and provision have pursued principles of equity and patient protection in their public policies on health services. The country case studies were selected in order to show that governments can have a legitimate interest in what goes on in the private sector and can reach very different accommodations between public and private interests in the health sector in the name of equity and patient protection. These experiences are then used in the last two chapters of the book to help develop proposals for improved regulation of public–private boundaries and relationships in UK health care in order to improve equity of access to services and patient protection.

References

1 Secretary of State for Health. *The NHS Plan: a plan for investment; a plan for reform.* Cm 4818-I. London: Stationery Office, 2000.
2 Burchardt T. *Boundaries between Public and Private Welfare: a typology and map of services.* London: London School of Economics Centre for Analysis of Social Exclusion, CASE paper 2, November 1997.
3 Burchardt T, Hills J, Propper C. *Private Welfare and Public Policy.* York: Joseph Rowntree Foundation, 1999.
4 Burchardt T. *Boundaries between Public and Private Welfare: a typology and map of services.* London: London School of Economics Centre for Analysis of Social Exclusion, CASE paper 2, November 1997.
5 Williams B. Utilisation of National Health Service hospitals in England by private patients, 1989–95. *Health Trends* 1997; 29: 21–5.
6 Ibid.
7 Department of Health. *Consultants' Contracts and Job Plans.* HC (90) 16. London: Department of Health, 1990: 2.
8 Light D W. The real ethics of rationing. *BMJ* 1997; 315: 112–15.
9 Audit Commission. *The Doctors' Tale: the work of hospital doctors in England and Wales.* London: Stationery Office, 1995.
10 Health Committee. *Consultants' Contracts.* Vol. I. Session 1999–2000, HC–586–I. London: Stationery Office, 2000: xi.
11 Doctors' and Dentists' Pay Review Body. *Twenty Eighth Report.* London: Stationery Office, 1998.

12 Audit Commission. *The Doctors' Tale: the work of hospital doctors in England and Wales*. London: Stationery Office, 1995.

13 Monopolies and Mergers Commission. *Private Medical Services*. Cm 2452. London: HMSO, 1994.

14 Yates J. *Private Eye, Heart and Hip*. Edinburgh: Churchill Livingstone, 1995: 90

15 Yates J, Harley M, Jayes B. Blade runners. *Health Serv J* 2000; 110 (5702): 20–3.

16 Ibid.

17 Propper C, Rees H, Green K. *The Demand for Private Medical Insurance in the UK. A cohort analysis*. Centre for Markets and Public Organisation Working Paper 013. Bristol: University of Bristol, 1999.

18 Ibid.

19 Yates J. *Private Eye, Heart and Hip*. Edinburgh: Churchill Livingstone, 1995: 108.

20 Bloor K, Maynard A. Rewarding health care teams. *BMJ* 1998; 316: 569.

21 Department of Health. *Agenda for Change: modernising the NHS pay system*. London: Stationery Office, 1999.

22 Secretary of State for Health. *The NHS Plan: a plan for investment; a plan for reform*. Cm 4818–I. London: Stationery Office, 2000.

23 Department of Health. *The NHS Plan – proposal for a new approach to the consultant contract*. London: Department of Health, 2001.

24 Salter B. The private sector and the NHS: redefining the Welfare State. *Policy Politics* 1995; 23: 17–30.

25 Office for National Statistics. *United Kingdom National Accounts (The Blue Book)*. London: Stationery Office, 2000.

26 Burchardt T, Hills J, Propper C. *Private Welfare and Public Policy*. York: Joseph Rowntree Foundation, 1999: 10.

27 Lewis R, Jenkins C, Gillam S. *Personal Medical Services Pilots in London – rewriting the Red Book*. London: King's Fund, 1998.

28 Calnan M, Cant S, Gabe J. *Going Private: why people pay for their health care*. Buckingham: Open University Press, 1993.

29 Ibid.: 91

30 Burchardt T, Hills J, Propper C. *Private Welfare and Public Policy*. York: Joseph Rowntree Foundation, 1999.

31 New B. The NHS: what business is it in? In: Harrison A, editor. *Health Care UK 1997–98*. London: King's Fund, 1998.

32 Parker R. Private residential homes and nursing homes. In: Sinclair I *et al.*, editors. *The Kaleidoscope of Care*. London: HMSO, 1990: 297–316.

33 Ibid.: 302.

34 Lewis J, Glennerster H. *Implementing the New Community Care*. Buckingham: Open University Press, 1996.

35 Royal Commission on Long-Term Care. *With Respect to Old Age*. Cm 4192–I. London: Stationery Office, 1999.

36 Secretary of State for Health. *The NHS Plan. The Government's response to the Royal Commission on Long-Term Care*. Cm 4818–II. London: Stationery Office, 2000.

37 Health Committee. *The Regulation of Private and Other Independent Healthcare*. Chapter 1. London: Stationery Office, 1999.

38 Hayward J. NHS dentistry. In: Appleby J, Harrison A, editors. *Health Care UK 1999/2000*. London: King's Fund, 1999: 98–107.

39 Taylor-Gooby P, Sylvester S, Calnan M, Manley G. Knights, knaves and gnashers: professional values and private dentistry. *J Social Policy* 2000; 29: 375–95.

40 National Association of Citizens Advice Bureaux. *Unhealthy charges: CAB evidence on the impact of health charges*. London: NACAB, 2001: 26–30.

41 Department of Health. *Modernising NHS Dentistry – implementing the NHS Plan*. London: Department of Health, 2000.

42 NHS Executive. *General Ophthalmic Services Activity Statistics, April 1999–September 1999*. London: NHS Executive, 2000.

43 New B. The NHS: what business is it in? In: Harrison A, editor. *Health Care UK 1997–98*. London: King's Fund, 1998: 178–97.

44 New B, Le Grand J. *Rationing in the NHS*. London: King's Fund, 1996.

45 Ibid.

46 Duncan A. Butler Memorial Lecture. 20 April 1999. Unpublished transcript of speech.

47 Hoffmeyer U K, McCarthy T. *Financing Health Care*. Amsterdam: Kluwer Academic, 1995.

48 World Health Organisation. *Life in the 21st Century – a vision for all*. WHO: Geneva, 1998.

49 Lea R. *Healthcare in the UK: the need for reform*. London: Institute of Directors, 2000.

50 Bosanquet N. *A Successful National Health Service*. London: Adam Smith Institute, 1999.

51 Secretary of State for Health. *The NHS Plan. The Government's response to the Royal Commission on Long-Term Care*. Cm 4818–II. London: Stationery Office, 2000.

52 Hoffmeyer U K, McCarthy T. *Financing Health Care*. Amsterdam: Kluwer Academic, 1995.

53 Judge K, Mulligan J-A, New B. The NHS; new prescriptions needed? In: Jowell R *et al.*, editors. *British Social Attitudes, the 14th Report: the end of conservative values?* Aldershot: Ashgate and SCPR, 1997: 49–72.

54 Blendon R, Leitman R, Morrison I, Donelan K. Satisfaction with health systems in ten nations. *Health Affairs* 1990; 9: 185–92.

55 HM Treasury. *Prudent for a Purpose. Working for a Stronger and Fairer Britain*. HC 346: Budget. London: Stationery Office, 2000.

56 Milburn A. *Reinventing Health Care. A Modern NHS versus a Private Alternative*. Speech at the London School of Economics. London, 20 December 1999.

57 Secretary of State for Health. *The NHS Plan: a plan for investment; a plan for reform*. Cm 4818–I. London: Stationery Office, 2000: 33–4.

58 Williams B, Whatmough P, McGill J, Rushton L. Patients and procedures in short-stay independent hospitals in England and Wales, 1997–1998. *J Public Health Med* 2000; 22: 68–73.

59 *Care Standards Act 2000*. Chapter 14. London: Stationery Office, 2000.

60 Ibid.

Chapter 5

Attempting to make private insurance equitable: the US experience

This is the first of two comparative chapters that attempt to contribute new experiences, perspectives and ideas to UK policy discussions about how the Government should strike the right public–private balance in health care, especially in the financial arrangements that underpin the relationships between public and private health services. At one end of this mix, there are countries that provide a universal and comprehensive health care system and prohibit a competing second tier. Somewhat less clear-cut are the arrangements in countries that provide a universal but less-than-comprehensive health care system, and which allow private care and financing to arise in the uncovered areas. For example, the Canadian system covers neither outpatient subscription drugs nor home health care, and the UK system no longer covers most long-term hospital care, dental care or optical services, except for the poor.

A variant of universal coverage is found in countries that use private insurance as an integral part of their universal health system (e.g. the Netherlands), rather than as a supplementary upgrade. Instead, private insurance provides the coverage of the public system for people above a certain income. The details of this are explained in Chapter 6.

Some countries, such as Canada, have not allowed private insurers or payers to offer coverage for the same services as the public system on more favourable terms.[1] The reasons for this arrangement are clear: if private insurers or payers are allowed to select only the more desirable, or popular, or profitable services in the universal system, this has the effect of creating two-tier access and weakens the underlying system. Furthermore, if only the healthier patients who can afford the premiums are selected, inequality of access increases further. Indeed, this describes the UK health care system – a universal service with private insurers and providers allowed to offer quicker access to selected services for selected subscribers, leaving the rest to be treated by the NHS. UK politicians and officials have for decades tended to behave as if private sector activity is beyond their purview and 'just happens' among those who want it. But supporting the private sector and two-tier access have been built into official health care policy from the beginning.[2]

An even larger role for the private sector is allowed in countries like Ireland that use private insurance extensively to compete with the public system and act as an upper tier of services. However, Ireland has worked hard to make this second tier as equitable and accessible as a second tier can be, and it provides an important model for how to set up competitive health insurance markets so that they reward efficiency and service rather than risk selection (*see* Chapter 6). This is difficult to achieve, because there are so many ways to 'game' the rules aimed at assuring equity and to win by insuring the easy risks, rather than by being more efficient or by providing better value for money.[3,4]

At the other end the spectrum, there are countries like the USA in which private insurance is the mainstay, and various public programmes take care of the millions who are too poor, too transient, too old, or too high risk to obtain cover. Such systems are explicitly two- or three-tiered.[5] In these systems, health care is a commodity, not a right, both in law and in fact.

We will start with the USA, because it illustrates most clearly the problems of a minimally regulated market in private insurance and the struggles by the State to cope with them. The US experience provides an object lesson for the UK. In the next chapter, we will turn to the Netherlands, where private insurers have played a major role alongside a publicly financed health care system, because the Netherlands highlights the boundary problems between public and private that persist, even within an egalitarian system. We will conclude with Ireland, because it has chosen to have a supplementary, top-up private insurance tier like the UK. Unlike the UK, however, it has developed as good a regulatory framework as any to protect the underlying publicly financed health service from being used by providers seeking private patients and by private insurers who want to cover only profitable services.

The US health care system – a public–private overview

The US health care system is by far the most complex in the world, and many powerful interest groups, including insurance companies, have spent years keeping it that way. As many observers have noted, this complexity has meant that few levers of control over expenditure, training, service mix, capital, major purchases, or geographical distribution have been possible or, if tried, effective.[6,7] An important complexity often not appreciated from abroad is that the Federal Government has no powers except for those specified by the Constitution; all other powers reside in each of the 50 States. Since the new Scottish Parliament and Welsh and Northern Ireland Assemblies have recently been formed in the UK, we shall pay some attention to the US experience of leaving most regulatory oversight to each State and the extensive obstacles this has created for establishing fair markets.

Private, risk-rated health insurance

The heart of US health care is a vast complex of private non-profit and for-profit provider groups, specialty clinics or centres, hospitals, home-health service corporations, surgical centres, and the like, covered under a wide variety of contracts with voluntary health insurance organisations and governmental agencies. We shall not attempt to describe the entire US health care system in all its complexity, but rather focus on those aspects of private insurance instructive for those concerned about its relationships with the public sector and the promotion of the social goals of equity and consumer protection.

US health insurance began when doctors and hospitals faced mounting piles of unpaid bills during the Great Depression of the 1930s. It was designed by the hospital associations and medical associations for acute, specialist care. It proliferated rapidly and became a standard benefit of employment in the decades after World War II.[8,9] Employer-based voluntary health insurance was the USA's answer to communist systems like the Soviet Union's and to 'socialist' systems like those in Germany or England.[10] It was based on the rhetoric of 'freedom and choice' – for doctors and hospitals, for employers and for subscribers. Since it was designed to reimburse what doctors and hospitals charged, private indemnity insurance fuelled the rapid expansion of costs with few controls. Today, US health care still costs about US$4000 per person each year, compared to the European average of about US$1700 and the UK average of about US$1300.[11] The US$4000 average per person includes 44 million people with no insurance who receive significantly fewer services. If they were to be given comparable access to needed services, without any other changes, the average cost would be even higher.

Employers choose (sometimes with the help of union representatives, but usually not) which services will be covered, how deep the coverage will be, the portion of the premiums that employees will pay ('co-premium'), the exclusion clauses for pre-existing conditions, how much employees must pay as a deductible initially, how much employees will pay of the bills thereafter ('co-pays'), and what limit will be set on these out-of-pocket payments. For example, a typical policy might require employees to pay 25 per cent of the premium, receive no payment for the first US$500 of bills (the deductible), face a nine-month exclusion clause for 'pre-existing conditions', and pay a 20 per cent co-pay for all bills up to a US$1200 ceiling (i.e. US$6000 of medical bills). (The term 'pre-existing conditions' refers to conditions that have started before a subscriber's policy begins to cover medical expenses. Conditions for which medical expenses are not paid include active illnesses or disabilities, but they usually include known risks, such as hypertension or being HIV-positive. With genetic profiling, the list of excluded conditions could expand considerably.) An example of shallow, but common, coverage would limit payments for outpatient mental health services to US$5000 a year and set a lifetime limit of US$30,000 for all mental health payments with, of course, no coverage for a pre-existing condition, such as depression, during the first nine months. A large secondary industry of health benefits consultants spends weeks helping employers custom-design their policies for fees of about US$3000 per day. Thus, a team of five consultants working with an employer for a month would cost US$300,000. From a provider's perspective, this employer freedom and choice results in thousands of policies with different terms of coverage and payment, using different forms. Administrative costs for designing and selling policies, for billing and monitoring services, and for running all the different parts of the US health care complex are very high, at about 25 per cent, or US$250 billion of more than US$1 trillion currently spent on health care.[12]

Social values and risk-rating

There are two basic concepts of justice that underlie health insurance.[13] Risk- or experience-rating is based on an ethic of *actuarial fairness*, which holds that it is unfair to force anyone else to pay for the health care costs of an individual's smoking or heart condition or greater age. That is, fairness should be based on actuarial risk alone. Competitive insurance markets accelerate risk-rating, because a chief way to lower premiums and thus win contracts is to risk-rate more finely, which is what has happened in the USA over the last few decades. Indeed, the logical endpoint of actuarial fairness is to have each sub-

subgroup (e.g. white males over 55 with a heart condition who smoke) pre-pay their costs in the form of premiums or receive lower coverage through treatment limits or exclusion clauses for pre-existing conditions, such as heart disease. By contrast, *social fairness* rests on the belief that a fair system provides access to needed services for everyone, and everyone should contribute equally or in proportion to their income. When these two ethics compete, as they do between private insurance in the UK and the NHS, *actuarial fairness always undermines social fairness*. That is, once some insurers are allowed to risk-rate, they naturally offer cheaper policies for the healthier members of a community-rated pool on which the pool depends to subsidise its sicker members. As this siphoning continues, the community-rated pool is forced to start risk-rating too or go bankrupt. In effect, insurance companies are investment funds that happen to cover risks. If their premiums approximately cover their costs, they still receive millions, or billions, of capital at no cost and invest it at a profit. The goal is to keep as much of the premiums as possible, for as long as possible, before having to pay as little as possible of the medical bills of subscribers.

Techniques of minimising risk and payments

Competing firms selling risk-rated policies can (and even *must*, to maintain or gain market share) elaborate risk-rating.

Table 5.1 lists the now-common forms of experience- or risk-rating by private health insurers in the USA.[14] They did not exist before employers became concerned about costs and pressed for the cheapest policies with no questions asked. Some of these techniques are probably used by health insurance companies in the UK, but no investigation has been made of their detailed practices when they bid for health insurance contracts from employers. All of the techniques are designed to minimise coverage of people with serious risks or health problems and to minimise payments for medical services (even though this is the opposite of what policyholders want them to do). Insurers in a competitive voluntary market have little choice but to follow the Inverse Coverage Law of unregulated health insurance: the greater one's medical needs, the less likely one is to obtain coverage for those needs and the more one is likely to pay for it.

The most common technique is to charge higher premiums to people who are older, or who exhibit a risk factor like high blood pressure, or who have an existing health problem or disease like depression or heart disease. The second

Table 5.1 The spiral of discrimination in risk-rated health insurance*

Techniques of Direct Risk-Rating

Traditional
    Charge higher premiums
    Insert exclusion clauses
    Deny coverage
    Red-line entire occupations or industries

Recent extensions
    Policy churning
    Within-group underwriting with exclusions
    Renewal underwriting
    Selective marketing

Techniques of Indirect Risk-Rating

Waiting periods
Deductibles
Co-payments
Payment caps
Benefits design

Techniques to Reduce Claims Paid

Increased co-payments, coverage limits and deductibles
Elaborated rules for validating claims ('gotcha' clauses)
Claims harassment
    Delayed responses
    No response
    Denial of valid claims
    Complex procedures, signature protocols, coordination of patient, physicians and facilities
    Unwritten internal rules of accounting
    Difficult forms to fill and responses to read
    Claims 'hot potato'
Exclusion by association
Phoney, fraudulent schemes
Pyramid schemes (take the money and run)
Policy switching

Source: Light D W. *JAMA* 1992; 267: 2503–8.

technique is to insert exclusion clauses that say, in effect, 'We will cover you except for medical expenses related to your diabetes.' A third technique is to deny coverage altogether, or not to offer policies in the first place to high-risk people. Exclusion clauses deny coverage for specific conditions or risks; denial means no coverage for any risk. A fourth technique, well-known in the UK, is long waiting periods for pre-existing conditions. There is good reason for a waiting period of up to one year for new subscribers, to prevent them from exploiting insurers (insurer moral hazard), but any longer time constitutes targeted denial of coverage of the health problems for which subscribers most need coverage. A fifth technique is to apply any, or all, of the others each year at renewal time, which is why many countries insist on guaranteed renewal of the same policy for the same premium, adjusted for an average increase in medical costs and perhaps for age. This common practice particularly offends long-time subscribers, who after 20 years of faithfully paying their premiums, get dropped when they are diagnosed with cancer. But, unless prohibited by law, each year is a new year and unrelated to the previous ones for private insurers. Finally, insurance companies in effect draw a 'red line' around certain occupations, a term that refers to banks 'red-lining' minority neighbourhoods where they will not sell any mortgages. Some US health insurers will not sell policies to anyone in a number of occupations deemed too risky. Some US insurers, ironically, list health care as an excluded industry. Why, indeed, should a sensible underwriter sell policies to people exposed to illnesses, infections and injuries every day, like nurses and doctors?

These techniques are slowly being taken up in the UK as private health insurance is becoming more competitive. Each company is forced to narrow the age and health-risk bands for a given policy, thus reducing the function of insurance, which is to spread risk over a wide group. Each is forced to charge higher premiums for those in higher-risk groups. If a company does not, it will lose money on its policies. As a second technique to hold down premiums, companies selling health insurance in the UK are reported to be quietly thinning out the coverage they provide and thus what they have to pay, through changes to their policies.

There are other, indirect ways to risk-rate, which are standard features in most health insurance policies (*see* Table 5.1). Waiting periods, deductibles, co-pays (user charges), and payment caps apply theoretically to everyone, but in reality they affect those with health problems, not the healthy. The design of benefits or pattern of coverage of a given policy, even on a level playing field of community-rating, can strongly shape the risk profile of the subscribers and how much of their medical bills get paid. Since most people do not know just what their health insurance policies cover, one recommendation is to require an up-front listing of everything that is *not* covered.

Recent extensions of the indirect risk-rating shown in Table 5.1 start with *policy churning*. In this technique, an employer changes insurers every year, so that the deductibles and the waiting period for pre-existing conditions start all over again. In this way, the employer stops paying medical bills for all new health problems, as well as for the old ones, which keeps the employer's premium low by not covering many of the medical needs of the employees. Another extension of traditional practices is to start writing exclusion clauses for employees with pre-existing conditions, known as *within-group risk-rating.*

Once subscribers need medical care, some insurance companies in the USA have found a number of ways to reduce the amount paid out – the third part of Table 5.1. Most of the techniques already mentioned for designing and selling policies reduce payout substantially. In addition, policies may have clauses that set conditions for validating claims, such as calling the insurer within 24 hours of a procedure, or submitting a bill within 30 days. Most subscribers have been found not to know about these requirements. Even if they do, as they are preparing for surgery or dealing with post-hospital recovery, they forget to follow the procedures and thus invalidate their bills for insurance payment. These are called 'gotcha' clauses in Table 5.1. The extent of their use in the UK is unknown.

The forms of 'claims harassment' listed in Table 5.1 are self-explanatory and very common. In the USA, there are few serious penalties for using them. For example, if insurance companies deny valid claims, a certain minority of subscribers will have the energy and resources to fight the denials and succeed in getting the claim paid several months or a few years later. But there are no penalties payable by the insurance companies. Meanwhile, the insurance companies can make daily interest on the funds retained. All delaying tactics like this can earn them months of additional investment income. Even regulations requiring that 'a valid claim be paid within 45 days' are easily circumvented by taking four, six or eight months to 'validate' the claim. The degree to which these practices are used in the UK is not known, though some hospital accident and emergency departments complain about not being paid for valid claims in relation to vehicle accidents.[15] The Health Committee took evidence of cases in which privately insured patients whose recovery ran into trouble were transferred to an NHS intensive care unit and displaced major elective surgical cases. Further, the bill for this expensive care was not paid.[16] In the USA, unpaid or delayed bills by insurance companies cause major financial problems for doctors and hospitals and create a great deal of administrative work. For patients, about 40 per cent of all personal bankruptcies are related to large uncovered medical bills.[17] To summarise, these direct and indirect techniques for minimising payments and discriminating against subscribers with illnesses, both when designing and selling policies and when handling claims, provide UK policy-makers with a list of practices they must address if they are to have fair markets in private health insurance.

'MediGap' – public–private interface and the failure of self-regulation

An instructive case of public–private relations and the difficulties of regulating private insurance in the USA occurred with respect to private insurance policies developed to pay for gaps in coverage in Medicare. Congress designed Medicare in the 1960s, with significant deductibles, co-pays, and coverage limits, in part because of the widespread belief at the time that user charges or out-of-pocket payments make patients more prudent users of health care and save money. Many studies have shown this belief to be erroneous. Patients do not shop or choose their health care except for low-cost initial visits, and if they are made to pay a considerable user charge, they reduce both unnecessary and necessary visits equally, with the latter leading to more expense when the medical problem finally gets treated. Beyond certain elective visits, patients are not the decision-makers, and user charges have perverse effects. Nevertheless, Congress decided to require patients to pay the first US$760 if they were hospitalised, US$95 a day after the first 20 days in a skilled nursing facility, all the costs of drugs not prescribed while in hospital, and 20 per cent of most outpatient medical services.[18] Private insurance companies soon discovered that the elderly did not want to be at risk for all these expenses and designed supplementary policies to fill these gaps in coverage.

Known colloquially as 'MediGap policies', they sold briskly, and then the complaints started pouring in. In the late 1970s, Congress investigated and the resulting testimonies provide one of the few inside portraits of marketing by commercial insurance companies.[19] They documented years of practices to avoid or reject sick elderly people, to sell policies with coverages already provided by the public programme, to sell duplicate policies, to sell policies with promised coverages that did not materialise, to sell a bewildering array of policies so that older people (who are otherwise experienced, frugal shoppers) could not comparison-shop, and to charge premiums far higher than the claims paid back. The health insurance industry calls the proportion of claims paid to premiums the 'medical loss ratio', a revealing term. Policyholders would call it the 'medical *benefit* ratio' if they controlled the language of insurance. Ratios were as low as 50 per cent, i.e. the insurance industry kept half of the premiums for administrative costs (including seven-figure executive incomes, marketing and profits). The industry lobbied hard to prevent Congress from passing regulations and promised to mend its ways on a voluntary basis.

Ten years then passed, and the same practices persisted, because they were so profitable and because individual companies would lose business if they tried to use them less than their competitors.[20,21] For these reasons, the health insurance industry finds it difficult to end such trade practices or discrimination on a voluntary basis. Any insurer who does so will put itself at a competitive disadvantage and lose market share to its competitors. Further, the industry itself is founded on underwriting and 'actuarial fairness', the opposite of social fairness.

Eventually, even cautious Congressmen lost faith in the ability of the health insurers to regulate themselves, and in 1990 Congress arranged to have standardised policies established, so that there could be a real market in which the elderly could compare prices. The regulations also set limits on the 'medical loss ratio'. Noting 'the extremely high incidence of fraud, misrepresentation and misinformation by agents',[22] Congress established rules to counter these practices. It prohibited any coverage that duplicated Medicare, and it established rules for the timely payment of claims and guaranteed renewal. An evaluation five years later found that the regulated market worked much better than before.[23] As we shall see in Chapter 6, the Dutch have established analogous rules.

However, insurance companies have found many ways to circumvent or neutralise such well-intentioned regulations. For example, they have handled the guaranteed renewal requirements set by Congress using the following strategies. First, they have simply raised premiums to unaffordable levels for patients with high risks or significant illnesses so that they 'choose' to drop their policies. As a consequence, these sick patients are forced into the open market as an uninsurable risk, which is exactly what 'guaranteed renewal' aimed to prevent. Meantime, some insurers regularly close blocks of policies as the policyholders get older and the claims mount, in order to leave the ageing and unhealthy risks in the closed block, set up a new block of business by filing and obtaining approval of a new policy form (usually at a premium rate that would attract the healthy new risks), and move the healthy risks from the closed block into the new block. Meanwhile, the insured in the closed block would, over time, experience the spiral of extreme premium rate increases coupled with the inability to find coverage elsewhere.[24]

From an international perspective, the Medigap story alerts UK and European policy-makers to several kinds of unfair trade practices that they need to avoid. These experiences, however, also indicate how difficult it is to deal with such practices. The Netherlands and Ireland (described in the next chapter) have come much closer to creating a level playing field than has the USA, even in this small, highly regulated segment of the US private insurance market. The UK has yet to identify a level playing field as a policy goal, perhaps because it regards the private medical insurance market as too small to be concerned about. However, as we have shown in earlier chapters, it does make a significant contribution to UK health care financing.

How well has risk-rated voluntary health insurance worked?

From a societal point of view, voluntary health insurance has created a number of problems. Its fragmented nature has prevented employers and society from using any of the strong levers of cost control enjoyed by most other industrialised democracies.[25] Competition drove costs up even faster than in previous periods, as providers and insurers strove to offer the most advanced equipment and the best specialist services. Coverage has become a serious problem, especially with the current push for cost containment. Recent reports document that less than 50 per cent of US employers now offer health insurance, and the premiums for individual policies for these workers on the retail market are extremely high.[26] The employer-based system is the primary insurer now for only 43.1 per cent of the US population.[27] The number of uninsured people has been rising at about 100,000 a month for nearly a decade, as employers have grown tired of the responsibility they assumed after World War II. The total uninsured population now stands at 44 million, or about one-sixth of the nation.[28] Three-quarters of these people are full-time workers or their dependants. Among poor workers, one-third have no health insurance to pay for medical bills.

Coverage among those who *are* insured is also thinning, as employers reduce their commitment.[29] Thus, employers who have provided health insurance to their employees are backing out of doing so, even though the economy and profits have been growing at record rates. The research office of Families USA estimates that a quarter of all Americans would have to pay 10 per cent or more of their income for uncovered medical bills if they became seriously ill or injured.[30] All forms of increased co-premiums, co-payments, coverage limits, payment limits and the like strongly discriminate against ordinary workers and the poor. This is because, first, each US$1000 paid for medical services is a greater proportion of their income, and second, they have more health problems than do middle-class people. These are consequences that might well result from decreasing the scope of coverage in the NHS and increasing the UK's reliance on private health insurance.

Beyond the failures of the voluntary health insurance market to provide good coverage at reasonable prices in an equitable manner is the pervasive commercialised atmosphere that develops. One notable recent example occurred when the Medicare administration became concerned that elderly people with serious mental health problems were not being followed up sufficiently intensively when they were discharged from hospital back to their communities. In response, administrators set up a programme for private mental health centres and psychiatrists to provide intensive outpatient care to these seriously disturbed elderly patients. The doctors and centres responded by seeing this as an opportunity to exploit the public programme. Billings to the new publicly financed programme soared, from an average of US$1642 per patient in 1993 to US$10,352 in 1997.[31] The number of centres quadrupled, from 250 to 1000. A Federal investigation found fraudulent claims in 91 per cent of the bills from the doctors and centres.

Regulating private health insurance

Given the long experience in the USA of establishing regulations for private insurance, it seems worthwhile to provide a brief and selective overview of issues and efforts that might help UK and European policy-makers learn from the experience.

At least half of US health insurance regulation concerns general insurance and started with the Insurance Company of North America, chartered in 1794.[32] Fair pricing has long been a general concern, especially since fire insurance companies in the 19th century often participated in co-operative rate-making in order to avoid 'the ruinous economic consequences … from unbridled rate competition'.[33] This is an example of insurance posing a classic dilemma for society. If rate competition is too fierce, it will drive insurers to risk their solvency, manipulate claims and customers, or perform other undesirable acts. But if there is co-operative rate-setting (which US anti-trust law prohibits), policyholders will pay more than they need to and competition will be undermined. Many States passed laws against co-operative pricing, but insurance companies found ways to circumvent them, e.g. by establishing 'advisory services' and setting rates co-operatively through them. This led to an alternative solution: to permit joint rate-making, but under the supervision of the State insurance commissioner. Most insurance commissioners, however, are appointed from the ranks of insurance company officers, and effectively this solution might give monopoly State power to a member of the club. To summarise, no clear solution to fair pricing in health insurance seems to have been discovered despite a century of efforts.

Fair prices and price-fixing have also been a focus of debate about whether the rules of insurance should be determined at the Federal or State level, a debate which seems germane to Scotland, Wales and Northern Ireland as they develop their own Parliaments and Assemblies. Originally, in the 19th century, the insurance industry supported bills for the Federal regulation of insurance companies, because they thought Federal regulation would be weaker than State regulation. However, the Supreme Court ruled in 1868 that even insurance policies sold across State lines were 'local transactions, and are governed by local law'.[34] By the 1930s, the industry had concluded that being subject to State laws gave it more focused influence and lobbying power in each of the States. Moreover, enforcement of insurance laws was weaker, since it tended to be carried out by understaffed, underfunded, and often undertalented State departments of insurance.

This arrangement was threatened when a regional underwriters' association, with officers from 198 companies, was indicted on the four counts of fixing rates, boycotting non-member companies and their agents, withholding patronage from purchasers of non-members, and withholding re-insurance facilities from non-members.[35] The State of Virginia Court dismissed the case because insurance was deemed to be regulated by individual States. However, in a 1944 landmark reversal, the US Supreme Court held that since insurance transactions crossed State lines, they constituted inter-State commerce. Furthermore, it held that Federal anti-trust laws applied. In response, insurance companies mounted efforts to exempt insurance companies from Federal anti-trust laws. They succeeded, and are today the only industry that can use the kinds of anti-competitive tactics, described above, with impunity. This tale may hold some lessons for the emerging Parliaments and Assemblies, and for Westminster.

Exemption from anti-trust laws was accompanied by various regulations requiring that policy changes should be publicly filed and that there should be public hearings and other safeguards. In practice, however, there are many ways in which insurance companies have breached or neutralised these safeguards aimed at making them act fairly and accountably. For example, premium increases have been *filed* publicly, but without any public notice, so that no one knew they had been filed. If an alert party noticed the filings and requested copies, they might not be made for six months, because the law only stipulated that requests be fulfilled, but not how quickly. Therefore, it appears from a review of the US experience since 1900 that insurance regulations should be detailed and national rather than broad and regional.

At the centre of thinking about insurance regulations is the question of whose interests should prevail, for the interests of consumers differ from the interests of insurers. Deciding this question determines, first, how laws are written, and second, how they are enforced. Once again, special measures are required if consumers' interests are to be represented and protected, starting with a well-paid and technically well-supported regulator to protect the vulnerabilities of policyholders and to protect insurers from unscrupulous policyholders. However, in the USA, the regulator who champions consumer interests, 'is apt to find himself out of office or precluded from finding a desirable berth in the industry after his term is over … Nor is the regulator likely to gain him useful support from the general public which is largely both inarticulate and uninformed in insurance matters'.[36] One exception was Herbert Denenberg, a distinguished professor of insurance who became a nationally known champion of consumers against the practices of insurance companies. He showed that a commissioner could translate actions and regulations into plain English, could talk with the Press and hold well-announced public hearings, and could force as much openness for consumers of insurance as consumers experienced when shopping for a car or a package holiday. Nevertheless, even the legendary Denenberg was forced to write:

> It is a sad and simple fact of life that the regulated provide a greater disciplinary force on the regulator than vice versa … The Commissioner is kept busy with brush fires and day-to-day encounters. He lacks the time and resources to take the long look … He is channelled into programs and dialogues the industry is interested in pursuing.[37]

Michael Dukakis, a Congressman who later became Governor of Massachusetts and a presidential candidate, wrote of the 'silent conspiracy' between regulators and the industry, which blocks needed reforms and stands in the way of consumer-oriented legislation: 'insurance departments have tended to become constituent agencies. Contact with the insurance industry is close and continuous'.[38] Even meetings of insurance commissioners were hosted by executives of insurance companies, and all press information was handled by publicists from major companies. Insurers, agents and brokers, Dukakis wrote:

> enact laws ostensibly in the public interest but actually in their own self-interest … Given a subject so recondite as insurance, it would be a singularly inept lobbyist who could not weave an aura of selflessness and public service about his client's predilections. No matter how conscientious, lacking adequate staff and consumed with other important matters, State legislators simply cannot cope with the spokesmen of these interest groups.[39]

More recent efforts to establish minimum standards of protection against free-market risk-rating have run into the same experiences. For example, Federal requirements to cover individuals with health conditions who pass four levels of eligibility failed to add 'at the same premium', and a 1999 US government study found that 90 per cent of insurance carriers charge a higher premium, with nearly half of them charging 300–364 per cent of the standard rate.[40] Most individuals with health conditions do not qualify for protection under the terms of the much-heralded Health Insurance Portability and Accountability Act of 1996 – a detail not usually mentioned. The study calls for closer monitoring of compliance, more consumer education, and similar measures that do not address either the loopholes in the law or the major circumventions by the insurance companies of its intent.

To conclude, this brief history of health insurance in the USA underscores the importance of establishing firm and detailed rules which reward insurance companies that provide better service and value, rather than reward techniques for minimising payment and coverage. The public–private issues have to do with establishing fair policies, markets and procedures for an industry in the USA that has resisted such efforts for over a century. The details given in this chapter illustrate the various pitfalls that need to be avoided if a country wishes to have fair markets and private health insurance that serves the public interest. UK private health insurance could benefit its customers and UK society, but only if the kinds of practices and problems identified here are properly addressed.

Thus, UK policy-makers need to ask themselves the following questions:

- Are the claims made by private insurers about the availability of NHS treatment (e.g. length of waiting times) accurate?

- Which health problems and treatments are covered and which ones are not covered in the private health insurance policies sold to individuals and employers?
- Are these coverages, their payments, and other terms (e.g. exclusions for pre-existing conditions or waiting periods) clearly expressed to potential subscribers? How well do policyholders understand them? Is it clear what is *not* covered?
- Which groups of prospective patients are effectively excluded from private insurance coverage, either because premiums are deliberately unaffordable or because coverage is refused?
- How prevalent are forms of claims harassment, 'gotcha' clauses, and other obstacles to getting claims paid?
- What scope for cost-shifting to the NHS do private policies allow? Do private insurers adequately compensate the NHS for the costs of care of patients transferred to the NHS due to complications encountered in the private sector?
- Is coverage of mishaps, complications and follow-up care required, so that patients and the NHS get the whole package of services for a problem paid?
- How easy or difficult is it to compare prices and policies? Are policies non-comparable as they often are in the USA?
- Are the policies priced fairly? Can one even tell? How effective are insurers' cost-containment methods from a patient perspective? What per cent of premiums is paid out in benefits? (It should be 80 per cent or higher.)

It is likely that no-one in the UK has the answers to these questions. A thorough survey of policyholders would be in order, as would a high-level review of options for structuring the market to benefit society. In the meantime, a few broad lessons can be drawn from experience in the USA.

1. Private insurance need not be as complex and costly as it is in the USA, but it has a natural tendency to become so because risk selection, coverage limits, exclusion clauses, the making of hundreds of non-comparable policies, and private pricing are highly profitable tactics. Increased competition in UK markets is forcing companies to differentiate their policies, thus making them more complicated. To avoid these, one needs simplifying rules that create a fair market in which a limited number of comparable policies are sold at open prices and without risk selection. Otherwise, the natural dynamics of competitive, commercial insurance are bound to increase these practices, as the affluent middle classes age and insurers find their costs rising. If one believes those experts who contend

that the NHS in its current guise is unsustainable,[41,42,43] then matters will get worse, although the Government's large cash injection for the NHS makes this less likely in the medium term. Fortunately, the OFT has become increasingly concerned about unfair trade and non-comparable health insurance policies in the UK, and the Financial Services and Markets Act 2000 will introduce substantial regulation of UK financial markets, and may well also strengthen oversight of key areas of private health care financing.[44,45] The question is whether the new legislation will be firm enough to require insurers to place a high value on consumer interests.

2. Providers are likely to exploit private insurers by charging high fees, and they can get quite aggressive about efforts by insurers to hold these high fees down to a reasonable level. A cycle of exploitation can quickly develop, as the insurers respond by charging still higher premiums to subscribers or by limiting their coverage in the various ways described above rather than attempting to manage clinician fees and costs directly. To avoid this widespread problem in Greater London and other cities, a fair *public* market in providers' charges needs to be set up so that wholesale and retail buyers (employers, insurers and patients) can shop for price and good value. This is already beginning to happen but needs full support, since it will be resisted by providers.[46]

3. For the sake of patients, as well as reducing potential exploitation of the NHS by private providers, Parliament needs to require that insurers and providers be clinically and financially responsible for follow-up care, mishaps, and complications surrounding a test or procedure. They must offer a package service for a package price. This is a better solution than the one recommended by the Health Committee, which seemed to focus heavily or solely on who should pay for intensive care if needed but did not provide a fair overall contract for individuals or employers who are paying the premiums.[47]

4. If private medical insurance is to avoid the pitfalls discussed in this chapter, from a societal point of view, a well-paid and technically well-supported regulator should be established both to protect policyholders from insurers and to protect insurers from unscrupulous policyholders.

Increasing attention is being paid to these issues in the UK. This is due in no small part to the work of the OFT, which has issued a series of increasingly firm reports, calling for stronger oversight of the design and selling of private medical insurance.[48,49] It appears that the industry has responded positively to some of the OFT's proposals, but has proved slow to provide full information to consumers about the nature and value of policies. It is a moot point whether the industry will respond more positively in the future. We will return to the work of the OFT, along with other regulators of financing and provision of UK health care, in Chapter 6. Before that, however, we consider in detail experiences in two other countries, the Netherlands and the Republic of Ireland.

References

1   Taylor M G. *Health Insurance and Canadian Public Policy*. Montreal: McGill-Queen's University Press, 1978.
2   Keen J, Mays N. Looking forward: will the fudge on equity sustain the NHS into the next millennium? *BMJ* 1998; 317: 66–9.
3   Light D W. The practice and ethics of risk-rated health insurance. *JAMA* 1992; 267: 2503–8.
4   Light D W. Life, death and the insurance companies. *New Engl J Med* 1994; 330: 498–500.
5   Reinhardt U E. A social contract for 21st century health care: three-tier health care with bounty hunting. *Health Economics* 1996; 5: 479–99.
6   Starr P. *The Social Transformation of American Medicine*. New York: Basic Books, 1982.
7   White J. *Competing Solutions: American proposals and international experience*. Washington, DC: The Brookings Institution, 1991.
8   Starr P. *The Social Transformation of American Medicine*. Book II. New York: Basic Books, 1982.
9   For a brief history, *see* Light, D W. The restructuring of the American health care system. In: Litman T J, Robins L S, editors. *Health Politics and Policy*. Third ed. Albany, NY: Delmar, 1997: 46–63. This volume contains many insightful essays about American health care by leading policy analysts.
10 'Communist' and 'socialist' are used here because these are the terms that have been widely used to characterise these systems in the USA.
11 Anderson G F. In search of value: an international comparison of cost, access and outcomes. *Health Affairs* 1997; 16: 163–71.
12 Woolhandler S, Himmelstein D U. The deteriorating administrative efficiency of the USA health care system. *New Engl J Med* 1991; 324: 1253–8.
13 Light D W. The practice and ethics of risk-rated health insurance. *JAMA* 1992; 267: 2503–8.
14 Ibid.
15 Eaton L. Intensive care doctors warn of non-payment by private insurers. *Health Service J* 1999; 1 April: 4.

16 Health Committee. *Regulation and Private Healthcare.* London: Stationery Office, 1999: Para. 131.

17 Gottlieb S. Medical bills account for 40% of bankruptcies. *BMJ* 2000; 320: 1295.

18 Bodenheimer T S, Grumbach K. *Understanding Health Policy: a clinical approach.* 2nd ed. Stamford, Conn: Appleton & Lange, 1998: Tables 2–3.

19 USA House of Representatives, Select Committee on Aging. *Abuses in the Sale of Health Insurance to the Elderly in Supplementation of Medicare: a national scandal.* Washington, DC: USA Department of Health, Education and Welfare, 052–070–04742–9, 1978.

20 McCall N, Rice T, Hall A. The effect of State regulations on the quality and sale of insurance policies to Medicare beneficiaries. *J Health Politics, Policy Law* 1987; 12: 53–76.

21 Shiles J L. *Medigap Insurance: proposals for regulatory changes and 1988 loss ratio data.* Washington, DC: USA General Accounting Office, 1990 (GAO/T-HRD-90-35).

22 National Association of Insurance Commissioners. *Medicare Supplement Insurance Minimum Standards Model Act: legislative history.* Kansas City: NAIC, 1995: 650–73.

23 Rice T, Graham M L, Fox P D. The impact of policy standardization on the Medigap Market. *Inquiry* 1997; 34: 106–16.

24 Ruch G. Medicare supplement simplification: myth or miracle. *J Ins Reg* 1993; 11: 466–75.

25 White J. *Competing Solutions: American proposals and international experience.* Washington, DC: The Brookings Institution, 1991.

26 Long S H, Marquis M S. *Trends in Offering Employer-sponsored Coverage.* Bulletin. No. 15. Washington, DC: Center for Studying Health System Change Data, 1998.

27 Carrasquillo O, Himmelstein D U, Woolhandler S. Going bare: trends in health insurance coverage, 1989–96. *Am J Public Health* 1999; 89: 36–42.

28 Rice D P. The cost of instant access to health care. *JAMA* 1998; 279: 1030.

29 Bodenheimer T, Sullivan K. How large employers are shaping the health care marketplace. *New Engl J Med* 1998; 338: 1003–7, 1084–7.

30 Shearer G H. *Hidden from View: the growing burden of health care costs.* Washington, DC: Consumers Union, 1998.

31 DePerle N M. Health care entrepreneurs seem to be alive and well. *New York Times* 1998; 30 September: 1.

32 Day J G. *Economic Regulation of Insurance in the USA.* 0-401-074. Washington, DC: USA Printing Office, 1970.

33 Ibid.: 18.

34 Ibid.: 15.

35 Ibid.: 23.

36 Ibid.: 63.

37 Denenberg H S. Insurance regulation: the search for countervailing power and consumer protection. *Insurance Law J* 1969; 556: 271–4.

38 Dukakis M S. The Hon. Legislators look at proposed changes. In: Keeton R, O'Connell J, McCord J, editors. *Crisis in Car Insurance*. Urbana: University of Illinois Press, 1968: 224.

39 Ibid.: 225.

40 USA General Accounting Office. *Private Health Insurance: progress and challenges in implementing 1996 Federal standards*. HEHS-99-100. Washington, DC: US General Accounting Office.

41 Bosanquet N. *A Successful National Health Service*. London: Adam Smith Institute, 1999.

42 Kanavos P. Economy and finance: a prospective view of the financing of health care. Report No. 5. In: Dargie C, editor. *Policy Futures for UK Health*. London: Nuffield Trust, 1999.

43 Lea R. *Healthcare in the UK: the need for reform*. London: Institute of Directors, 2000.

44 Office of Fair Trading. *Health Insurance*. London: OFT, 1996.

45 Office of Fair Trading. *Health Insurance*. London: OFT, 1998.

46 Richards T. Educator with a vision. *BMJ* 1999; 319: 146.

47 Health Committee. *The Regulation of Private and Other Independent Healthcare*. 281-I, Session 1998–99. London: Stationery Office, 1999: Para. 132.

48 Office of Fair Trading. *Health Insurance*. London: OFT, 1998.

49 Richards T. Educator with a vision. *BMJ* 1999; 319: 146.

Chapter 6

Two forms of public–private health insurance partnership

If the US experience provides an instructive catalogue of tactics used by private insurers in a minimally regulated market to discriminate against those most in need of coverage and to frustrate fair trading practices, the Dutch and Irish experiences provide an instructive catalogue of efforts to develop and maintain a much more equitable legal framework that treats private health insurance as an integral part of the overall health care system. Both the Dutch and Irish systems aim to provide universal access to a comprehensive range of services that are largely free at the point of service. However, private insurance in Ireland constitutes a widely used second tier of privately financed access, which is about as equitable as a second tier can get. By contrast, private insurance in the Netherlands is an integral and equitable part of the wider health care system and not primarily a second, higher tier. Both countries provide fresh perspectives and useful ideas for current UK policy debates.

The Netherlands: blending private and public health insurance equitably

The health care system in the Netherlands reflects the principles of solidarity, universal access and equal treatment, professional autonomy and cost control. The tensions between these principles and the resolutions between them have formed the dynamics of policy over time.[1] These principles are similar to those in the UK, but the means for putting them into practice and financing them are quite different. Whereas the UK NHS is funded predominantly from general taxation collected by central government, and the majority of its services are delivered through hospitals and other provider organisations owned by the State, the Dutch system is funded through a mixture of mandated and voluntary forms of health insurance, from public, private but non-profit, and for-profit insurance funds or companies, and services are delivered largely by private, non-profit providers.[2,3] The Dutch system represents a paradox for most outside observers: one of the most equitable and universal systems, with minimal contributions from the Government or from patients' pockets, yet developed in a country that has consistently opposed proposals for national health insurance.

The three components of Dutch health care financing

The Dutch financing system is composed of three components:

- a foundation of government-financed coverage for long-term care, catastrophic costs and other 'non-insurable' costs and patients, such as the chronically ill or disabled
- mandatory coverage for people earning below an income ceiling
- private voluntary insurance for those with higher incomes or working for government.

Underpinning both the mandatory sickness funds and voluntary private insurance is the AWBZ,* the long-term and exceptional expenses insurance scheme. Started in 1968 as a population-wide safety net of social insurance, this universal programme has expanded from covering long-term institutional care to include home care, supported living accommodation for the physically and mentally handicapped, inpatient and outpatient rehabilitation, extended mother and child care, vaccinations, prenatal testing and other services. These extensions have increased the AWBZ's share of total health care expenditure from 25 per cent in 1989 to 38 per cent in 2000.[4] Funds are raised through income tax for the first step of taxable income, at 10.25 per cent. In addition, there are considerable user charges, though income-related, which constitute 11 per cent of all expenditure for AWBZ services. The critical effect of the AWBZ is to remove high risk from all other health insurance policies, so that even people who depend on a private insurance policy to pay their medical bills are not at serious risk.

The second component – mandatory health insurance by the sickness funds – covers 63 per cent of the population but pays for only 37 per cent of health care costs because of the existence of the AWBZ. Legally defined coverage for the funds includes the cost of most acute medical care, prescription drugs, medical aids and appliances, brief physiotherapy, speech and occupational therapy, home dialysis, some related services, and dental care for young people. The funds are both publicly- and privately-run insurance organisations that receive their budgets from a Sickness Fund Council, into which employers and employees pay a fixed per cent of their wages. In 2000, the rates were 1.75 per

---

* Algemene Wet Bijzondere Ziektekosten 1967 (Exceptional Medical Expenses Act 1967).

cent and 6.35 per cent respectively of employees' income, up to a cap of 55,900 guilders. The Council sets budgets for individual funds and supervises them. Although these budgets once reflected the sum of bills submitted for treatments and reimbursed, they are now prospective and risk-adjusted by age, gender, region, and disability status.[5] Since 1999, sickness funds have been responsible for all of their over-spending on the variable costs of services used by their subscribers. Sickness funds receive separate payments for capital investments and for the excess costs of certain high-risk groups. The funds, in turn, contract with providers and facilities for their services, increasingly in a proactive manner as cost-conscious purchasers. Over time, the sickness funds have consolidated from more than 1000 before 1940 to about 88 in the mid-1980s, and 30 in 1999. Six of them account for over 60 per cent of sickness fund enrolees.[6]

The third component, voluntary private health insurance, is available to the 36 per cent of Dutch residents above the income ceiling for sickness fund insurance and can be offered either by an insurance company or by the sickness funds as an adjacent product line. Almost everyone above the income ceiling has private health insurance, though it is not compulsory, choosing from a variety of policies and usually getting at least the same coverage as that provided by the sickness fund policies. Although private health insurers 'are free to determine premiums, coverage and underwriting practices',[7] the range of practices is quite modest for historical, political and cultural reasons explained below. Overall, they account for 14 per cent of expenditure.

Applicants for a private policy must fill out a detailed application and medical history, and policies are risk-rated, largely in terms of higher deductibles. Premiums are increased for all policyholders. There is some risk discrimination during the waiting periods and exclusion clauses, and private policies may have user charges on specific services or items, such as prescription drugs. However, many Dutch policy-makers feel that user fees are not worth the trouble and expense of collection. They can lead people with modest or low incomes to avoid taking medicines or seeing a clinician when they should. Once a person subscribes, renewal of a policy is guaranteed. Many people obtain their private insurance through employer-sponsored collective contracts, and while group policies are risk-rated, Dutch insurers have not employed the more aggressive or discriminatory techniques found in the USA, such as within-group risk-rating.[8] The policies are also 'portable', i.e. they can be continued even if one changes employers.

Out-of-pocket expenses total less than 7 per cent of health care costs. Compared to other European countries, Maarse and de Roo observe that nowhere is the proportion of cash payments so low, and nowhere is the proportion of private insurance so high.[9] Yet nowhere is private health insurance so fully integrated into the social goals of the overall system and plays so little of its typical role as a second-tier upgrade for the better-off.

As well as these three basic components and cash payments, there are supplementary health insurance policies. In recent years, private insurers have collaborated or merged with sickness funds to expand their markets for selling these policies. About half of sickness fund members have purchased additional coverage, but unlike private health insurance in the UK, this coverage is prohibited from duplicating coverage in the main policies, so that two-tier access can be minimised. Neither private nor supplementary policies can be used by patients for jumping Dutch waiting lists or for supporting a private, side business that specialists typically build up on the back of the universal system, as they do in the UK. Thus, supplementary private policies are limited to additional benefits beyond the social insurance scheme, in the same way as private supplemental policies function in Canada and among the elderly in the USA under Medicare.

For example, it is possible to buy policies that pay for user fees, especially for AWBZ services for patients with good incomes, or for extended services, such as more comprehensive dental care. Supplementary policies, for example, can allow one to move from a three-to-six-bed hospital room to a two-bed or single room, or a single room with a minibar, fax, computer, fresh flowers and other extras. Yet few hospitals have developed such facilities on the grounds that there appears to be little demand for them. Moreover, most patients are assigned to a hospital room based on their medical problem, not their hotel preferences, and when they get lower-grade accommodation than their supplementary policy entitles them to, they are paid a rebate as compensation. In such ways, the private market for supplementary policies is not allowed to undermine equity very seriously, and Dutch people as a whole seem to agree that more affluent people should be able to pay for upgraded accommodation or extra services but not for better or quicker medical care. Thus, Dutch law, regulations and administrative practices may provide a valuable resource for any policy-makers in the UK or elsewhere who wish to make private health insurance both more equitable in its own right and less threatening to the mainstream system. However, one can see potential lines of tension in these finely tuned arrangements: for example, for waiting lists and times lengthening, or for more new procedures not being covered by policies. Currently, there is pressure from employers who want to reduce their costs for sick pay by having employees on waiting lists treated privately right away.

Finally, the Government pays for public health services, such as screening and other preventive measures, out of general taxes. The public health package is becoming more comprehensive as the country recognises the increasing role of prevention for maintaining health and containing costs. The Government also subsidises university hospitals and, to a small extent, supports the compulsory and voluntary insurance schemes as well. Government direct funding, however, accounts for only 5 per cent of health spending. In short, the Dutch have developed, step by step, in response to emerging needs and perceived inequities, universal access and coverage for a range of services more comprehensive than that provided by the UK NHS, yet with very little direct government funding.

This interesting scheme of three major and three minor financing components warrants reflection. The public–private Dutch health care system centres on establishing *boundaries* that can be changed, between public and private, between solidarity and individual choice, and between equity and choice. The public components and state control have grown over time, largely in response to inequities in the private sector. The solidarity principle holds that contributions should be income-related, although overall they are slightly regressive. Adverse selection is prohibited, though it is inherently present in private insurance. The universal safety net for long-term and exceptional costs, the AWBZ, assures provision for the cost-effective management of chronic conditions, rehabilitative care, costly long-term care and certain preventive measures. The scheme could be expanded progressively so as to become, in effect, a universal health insurance scheme. Yet doing this is regarded as too radical, and proposals for universal health insurance have been voted down as too 'socialistic'. Likewise, the income ceiling for mandatory participation in the sickness funds could be raised ever higher, so that the sickness fund policies, together with the AWBZ, would constitute a universal public health insurance scheme. That has slowly happened to an extent. The background to these options and how the system developed can deepen our understanding of policy options that might be usable elsewhere.

Managing contested boundaries between countervailing powers

The history of the Dutch health care system, like all health care systems, involves the assault on, protection of, and negotiation of *boundaries by countervailing powers*. Although the concept of countervailing powers was first developed by Galbraith[10] to describe market dynamics, it can be used to analyse the medical profession in its dealings with the State, major payers, patients, and insurers.[11] In the Dutch case, the countervailing powers included the sickness funds, private insurers, the organised professions, and the State as both referee and the rules committee overseeing the contested terrain. A brief history of Dutch health insurance neatly illustrates several boundary issues between countervailing powers; one such contest might be called 'the taming of private health insurance'.

In the early 20th century, sickness funds were developed by unions, employers and mutual-aid societies to protect workers from income loss due to injury or illness. According to Schut, these funds largely covered the costs of seeing the doctor and drugs: 'Providing financial access to hospital and specialist care was traditionally left to municipal goverments and later also to local hospital insurance funds.'[12] The funds found doctors willing to sign cheap capitation contracts for services, which meant they passed most of their risk on to the doctors. Small private health insurance companies arose to offer more affluent citizens reimbursement for GP visits, drugs and hospital care, with providers setting their own fees and charges. Private insurers applied stringent underwriting practices and provided limited coverage. Thus, these two sets of organisations embodied two quite different approaches and values. One aimed to help members get medical care at the lowest possible cost on a non-profit, mutual basis, while the other aimed to support private practice and make money by selecting lower-risk private subscribers.

The organised medical profession represented a third force, centred on developing top-quality clinical medicine, professional autonomy and private practice. Fearing that the sickness funds might expand their low-pay policies into the middle classes, the Dutch Medical Association closed ranks in 1912, by requiring that doctors were only to contract with the funds for patients below a specified low income. Public provisions and low-cost care were acceptable to doctors for patients who could not afford private fees, but not for those who could. This monopolistic move in protection of their incomes echoed similar but more militant initiatives in Germany by its private medical practitioners.[13]

Ironically, the eventual harnessing of private health insurance to larger social goals took place with the invasion of the Netherlands by Hitler's army.[14] The German occupiers imposed a three-part structure in the Sickness Funds Decree of 1941:

- compulsory health insurance for wage earners and dependants below a working-class wage level
- voluntary insurance for non-wage earners
- private voluntary insurance for the rest.

The Decree required the funds to include hospital-related expenses, to use community-rating and have open enrolment, so that this level of social justice increasingly became the norm. The deficits of sickness funds were pooled and reimbursed by the Government. These changes strengthened sickness funds and raised their status to a mainstream social institution. As an unanticipated consequence, they could now cross the line into private health insurance. Since sickness funds paid relatively low fees and had administrative costs about half those of private insurers, their premiums were lower, even though they were required to have open enrolment and use community-rating rather than select risks and charge accordingly. As a result, the sickness funds established related subsidiaries and offered competing policies to the private sector. This also allowed them to keep their subscribers as their incomes rose above the limit for mandatory coverage by selling private policies without the marketing costs of soliciting new business. Their market share rose from 8 per cent in 1950 to 40 per cent in 1959 at the expense of the private insurers.[15]

In response, a number of private insurers formed a cartel in 1957 in order to counter these developments and address the inherent weaknesses of competition. This irony is often overlooked: namely, that competition amongst private health insurers leads them to intensify their search for better risks (as the easiest way to maximise profits and minimise losses), but that this, in turn, increases their transaction costs for searching, marketing and monitoring.[16] These natural forms of competitive behaviour alienate customers, the public and politicians, who can nationalise them ultimately or eliminate them altogether. By acting in concert, however, private insurers set limits or boundaries to their own competitive practices. They agreed to:

- guarantee the renewability of policies held regardless of how policyholders' health changed

- increase premiums for everyone equitably rather than just for those at higher risk
- cover all new babies regardless of risk
- limit the use of exclusion clauses for pre-existing conditions
- establish a re-insurance pool for high-risk subscribers.

Although its premiums were higher, the pool protected private insurers from the dangers of enrolling disproportionately high-cost patients. This pool was improved over time. These self-imposed efforts to set limits on competition worked. Private health insurance policies became more stable and attractive, and the public came to trust them. As a result, more citizens took out policies, and the percentage of the voluntary private sector who subscribed rather than paid cash for services rose from 72 per cent to 92 per cent.[17] Broad policy coverages and community-rated underwriting practices became increasingly standardised.

This sequence of events contradicted classical economic theory but fitted historical and institutional approaches in economic sociology to explain economic behaviour. Contrary to economic theory, commercial insurers did not attempt to regain market share by refining risk-rating or targeting low-risk groups as they did in the USA during the 1960s and 1970s (*see* Chapter 5).[18] Despite much more refined actuarial data and information technology, 'the cartel of commercial health insurers was unwilling to exploit this opportunity'.[19] They feared that social and political expectations would have prompted regulatory action if they had done so. Worse, they would have had to raise premiums for their older subscribers as they lowered them for low-risk subscribers, offending the public even more and perhaps even prompting politicians to universalise the sickness fund scheme so that private health insurance would be eliminated. In fact, the Government introduced a proposal for national health insurance in 1975. It did not pass into law but it manifested the danger to the industry if it did not impose effective self-restraint. The rules committee (the State) could remove them from the field.

Rapidly escalating costs in the 1970s, however, destabilised these arrangements, because the relative advantage to new insurers of offering lower-priced policies to low-risk subscribers was so great. An increasing number of insurers introduced community-rated policies with high deductibles to attract low-risk individuals. This strategy was less visible and therefore less politically provocative than lowering premiums, and it was more effective in driving out high-risk subscribers. Initially, it also avoided what Schut accurately calls the 'deadly premium spiral' that occurs when new insurers offer lower premiums to lower-risk subscribers, thus drawing them away from the older insurers, thereby leaving them with proportionately higher costs and lower income.[20] The older insurers must compete by lowering their premiums, but this of course means their losses are even greater. There is no way out. High-deductible policies are not quite so deadly or direct as low-premium policies, but as they rose from 3 per cent in 1971 to 84 per cent in 1978 of all policies, high-risk patients became the victims.[21] Fortunately, they could move across to the sickness fund voluntary policies, but as they did, they created a crisis of adverse selection in those funds. Their community-rated premiums had to increase, which induced young low-risk subscribers to leave, making the risk imbalance even worse and creating a 'fatal premium spiral' for the sickness funds. According to Okma, 'This marked the end of community-rating, and the start of a spiralling process of risk selection and premium differentiation. It also ended the existing solidarity between the healthy and the sick, and between the young and the elderly ... Insurers started to exclude pre-existing conditions from coverage.'[22] To compete with the new 'cream-skimming' insurers, old-line insurers broke with tradition and introduced age-related premiums. Other insurers had to follow suit, as the premium death spiral quickened.

The insurers tried to address these problems in 1983 by introducing a voluntary form of pooling high-risk expenses and reducing the differences in age-related premiums. 'However, the voluntary pooling efforts failed, causing internal conflict between the private insurance companies. Efforts to solve the problems through self-regulatory measures had little or no success. The patience of the Cabinet waned, and Parliament lost its faith in the self-regulatory powers of the private insurance world.'[23] The voluntary funds turned for relief to the Government, which more than doubled its subsidies to keep the funds afloat.

The Government was determined to strengthen regulation of the private insurance market pending a more fundamental restructuring of health care finance for managed competition (which never happened).[24,25] It passed the WTZ, or Health Insurance Access Act, which terminated the voluntary sickness fund scheme and required private insurers to offer enrolees comprehensive benefits for legally determined premiums. Resulting deficits were pooled and the deficit paid by imposing a flat charge or 'tax' on the subscribers. Thus, public intervention reset the boundaries and terms of private insurance policies and companies, which had shown that they were no longer entirely able, in the high-cost world of modern medicine, successfully to maintain equitable markets through self-regulation.

Financial access for the privately insured elderly, however, continued to worsen because of risk segmentation by insurers and the rising costs of specialty medicine. For example, the hospital costs of privately insured men over 80 years old increased from 4.9 times the costs of men aged 45–49 years to 7.6 times greater. Legislators intervened again in 1989 to amend the WTZ so that all people over the age of 65 below a certain income became eligible for the cross-subsidised standard policies. In 1991, the WTZ was further amended to allow all people with private insurance paying more than the standard policy to exchange their policy for the standard one. These measures did not go as far as national health insurance and yet reduced many of the problems associated with a private insurance market. Meanwhile, the opposite problem was happening to students. Due to community-rating, they had to pay considerably more than their low risk warranted; yet their low incomes made such policies unaffordable. The solution was to give them access to standard policies at very low rates. Another problem was that low-earning, self-employed people had to pay proportionately higher premiums for private insurance plus the two flat-rate mandatory 'contributions' – one within private insurance and one between private insurance funds and sickness funds. This was also considered too unfair, so they are now eligible for sickness fund insurance, irrespective of their incomes.

Besides strengthening the arrangements for risk-pooling *within* the private insurance sector through legislation, the Government has created forms of cross-subsidisation *between* the private insurers and the compulsory sickness funds, because the sickness funds attracted a disproportionate number of older and chronically ill people because they tended to have lower incomes. Subscribers to private health insurance now pay a second set of flat-rate contributions to compensate the sickness funds for their over-representation of older people and those with chronic illnesses. In these ways, inequities in private health insurance have been addressed, one by one, by different governments over many years.

Another boundary has gradually shifted during these decades, with profound consequences for access and quality. Mandatory sickness fund coverage was traditionally limited to the poor and lower-working classes. Given that the funds paid doctors and hospitals poorly, while private insurance reimbursed fees and charges, a strong two-tier system of services developed. By the 1960s and even into the 1970s, private insurers paid as much as four times the amount that sickness funds paid to specialists. Doctors had separate waiting rooms for sickness fund and private patients, and they scheduled separate hours with them. Sickness fund patients were more likely to be seen by a junior doctor, while private patients were more likely to be seen by the senior specialist. Gradually, however, the income ceiling for eligibility to the sickness funds has been raised, and this boundary shift has slowly altered the culture of the funds as they increasingly represent the middle classes. It would be as if Medicaid in the USA went from covering half of the very poor to all of the working class and then much of the middle class. The current income cap for mandatory coverage is 65,000 guilders, a respectable middle-class income. As the ceiling was raised, the traditional discrepancies between the two classes of care came under increasing cultural and political pressure. Private insurance reimbursement to providers decreased to three times as much, then twice as much, and finally the same as sickness fund pay when, in 1995, the COTT or Central Organisation for Payments in Health Care equalised how providers were (and are) paid. Recently, an expert explained that the amounts providers are paid no longer depends on what type of health insurance a patient has. This development also harnessed private health insurance to the larger social goals of equitable health care. Most relevant for the UK, private insurance is not, and cannot be, used to jump waiting list queues. Insurers can, and do, have initiatives to shorten waiting times, but they are aimed at all clients.

Thus, the Netherlands has a large private insurance market, but one strongly and increasingly harnessed to egalitarian goals of access and service in response to the natural tendencies of private insurers to discriminate repeatedly against those with high risks, when these are the people who most need coverage. Such tendencies led Light to characterise private health insurance as ruled by the Inverse Coverage Law: the more one needs good health insurance coverage, the less likely are private insurers to provide it and/or the more they will charge for it.[26]

The harnessing of private insurance to fulfil more egalitarian social goals has occurred at three levels:

- the cultural level of changing expectations and values, leading to institutional changes and boundary negotiations
- the collective voluntary level of insurers disciplining themselves
- the regulatory level of the Dutch Parliament and the Ministry of Health establishing laws and administrative regulations.

Regarding the second level, although Dutch and EU laws now prohibit the older, cartel-like measures (even if done to benefit society), Dutch insurers still volunteer to accept and cover all newborn children under standard terms. They also include guaranteed renewability clauses in their policies, thus limiting themselves to raising premiums for higher-risk policyholders at renewal time, but not dropping them.

The risk-pooling arrangements created by the Dutch legislature and Government demonstrate the complexity of reconciling actuarial justice with social justice,[27,28] or what Europeans call 'the equivalence principle with the solidarity principle'. Very few countries have done it so well as the Dutch, and it has taken decades of controversy and compromise, a warning to others that they may not do it so well. Private insurance is based on the principle that people with similar risks should be treated alike and that it is unfair to make people with lower risks pay for those with higher risks at a population level. By contrast, social insurance is based on the principle that the healthy should subsidise the less healthy and that everyone should make the same community-rated contributions. In recent years, community-rating has been refined to address the problem of premiums being too expensive for young people, when it is vital to get them into any broad community-rated pool.[29,30]

On the provision side, most Dutch health care is private and non-profit. Hospitals, clinics, home-care agencies and such like are all private. Specialists are private practitioners who have traditionally charged fees for services, though increasingly they are being paid salaries. In either case, the budgets for their services have been integrated with their hospital budgets so that they share responsibility for keeping hospital-related expenses within budget. However, this major decision locks specialists into hospitals and locks health care budgets into hospitals, thereby erecting obstacles to developing intermediate and integrated services with primary care, which is provided, as in the UK, by GPs who receive a *per capita* budget and who serve as the gatekeepers and co-ordinators for specialist services. This system of private provision is heavily regulated and supervised by state planners. To put it another way, the borders of private provision are heavily patrolled. But as Maarse and de Roo point out, the publicly regulated system also absorbs, and even invites in, new private providers by permitting them to become certified and affiliated with mainstream providers.[31]

Problems of a segmented system

The existence of public and private sources of funding, some of which are income-related and some not, operating on different social and moral principles and using different methods of financing in a society that values highly equity and access, produces a number of policy problems that are legion in the USA but largely ignored. These problems are widely shared in systems throughout the world using 'Bismarck-type' insurance schemes, but are largely unknown in the UK. Nevertheless, they are instructive to any consideration of managing the public–private mix in health care and to issues raised by any potential expansion of the role of private insurance.

From this account of the Dutch health insurance system, one can see how the two major public components have been built up to address injustices and inadequacies in the private component, and how private health insurance has been integrated into an overall national system. But this still leaves the Dutch with a segmented system and constant boundary problems. What should be the upper limits of income above which people should cover their own medical expenses? What boundaries between choice and inequity should be set regarding what policies should and should not cover? Other problems have to do with people or cases at the boundaries. For example, someone earning just below or above the cut-off income for voluntary health insurance may end up paying an unfair excess. Such boundaries involve obligations and relationships, as well as a range of choice and degree of inequity. Moreover, there is constant pressure to allow more inequity into the system or, in the other direction, to allow more options and choice for the increasing number of affluent citizens as they age.

One obvious solution that keeps reappearing is to eliminate private health insurance altogether, except for supplementary policies. The AWBZ could be expanded to cover everything, or mandatory insurance could be expanded to cover everyone. Or both could be combined into a national health insurance scheme covering nearly everything, with 5–15 per cent of costs at risk, as proposed in the late 1980s to promote managed competition. So far, the Dutch have done none of these and their problems remain. Separate insurance schemes for acute and long-term care can (and do) lead to cost-shifting from one budget to another in the case of patients with expensive health problems. They also frustrate or even prevent more efficient designs of services that can reduce costs for both schemes by providing forms of intermediate care integrated with primary care. By contrast, current UK policy aims to make primary care organisations responsible for developing integrated services by giving them the budget to do it. This, or any similar proposal, would be nearly impossible to execute in the Netherlands because of the segmented insurance structure.

Segmented service contracts are another obstacle to more cost-effective services, and are found in many health care systems. The problem centres on very large contracts with acute hospitals and sometimes with long-term institutions as well. These institutions are typically the organisational and budgetary homes for specialists as well. Yet the innovations of modern medicine and equipment permit more cost-effective and flexible configurations of services that can respond to the changing clinical needs of patient groups, with hospitals as a last resort rather than the main port of call.[32] Segmented contracts prevent any of this happening, and the Dutch decision to tie specialists even more firmly into hospitals adds a further obstacle to developing patient-centred, cost-effective services through integrated service contracts between primary care organisations and specialists.[33]

More choice? Less equity?

In theory and in practice, Dutch patients have quite a bit of choice. They can choose their GP, and they have a good deal of say about the specialists, hospitals and other providers they use. But there is pressure for more choice, especially in terms of service upgrades. The equalising of pay and services between patients with voluntary private or mandatory insurance may have raised services for the latter, but it has also equalised services at a certain level. Suppose, for example, you are in a standard Dutch nursing home. Accommodation is adequate in your four-bedded room, and the food is acceptable; but you're there for the long haul, and you want to pay for a private room with interesting and delicious food. You do not have that choice. The nursing home is not set up to make this provision. As a result, things are changing. Private companies are building upscale nursing homes for affluent clients. Then the question will be, what does the public pay for, and what does the patient pay for privately? The easy and perhaps most likely answer will be that patients (or their supplementary insurance policies) will pay for upgrades beyond a decent standard. But at the same time, more choice is being built into public provision as well.

The most notable experiments are in AWBZ long-term and home care. Patients now have to be assessed by an independent agency to determine what their needs are and what services the AWBZ will pay for, which is itself a public–private boundary management measure. But it is now proposed that the AWBZ simply gives patients the budget for their care and lets them decide how they want to organise and get it. Once they decide, they can order the AWBZ to pay the bills, up to the limit of their allocated budget. This would provide a great deal more private choice than has ever been possible before, yet within the budgetary limits of public insurance.

The confluence of choice and competition to contain *government* costs centres on regarding the AWBZ, the sickness funds, and supplemental policies as three 'compartments' of the same funding system.[34] With the AWBZ as a national base, competition has been introduced into the second compartment by allowing sickness funds to compete across regions, to be free from the obligation to contract with every provider, and to set their flat-rate top-up premiums as they see fit. So far, these major policy changes have produced little change on the ground, but it is early days, and sickness funds are not yet at risk for all of their variable payments to providers. But it is the supplemental private insurance policies that are 'becoming an increasing point of leverage as the government tries to reduce the scope of benefits in the second component'.[35]

The new waiting lists

Waiting lists for elective acute care along the lines of the UK NHS are a relatively recent phenomenon in the Dutch system and seem to be an unanticipated consequence of other policy changes. One change was to stop reimbursing specialists and hospitals for their bills and instead give them risk-adjusted population-based budgets. A second was to end the regional monopolies that sickness funds had enjoyed for years and to foster greater competition among them. They, too, have risk-adjusted population-based budgets, putting further pressure on holding down expenses in order to keep premiums competitive. A third policy change was to end the two-tier higher payments and services for patients with private insurance (*see above*). These changes have led to hospitals being unable to treat every patient referred and even running out of money. Waiting times have become a serious issue. Maarse and de Roo point out that this has caused bottom-up pressure for change that is quite different from the previous top-down proposals for reform.[36] Now patients and specialists are advocating competition as a possible solution to the budgetary–waiting time squeeze. Furthermore, a fourth recent policy change has made employers financially responsible for the extended sick-leave pay of their workers. We have heard that some employers are contracting with private providers outside the system to treat their employees rapidly and get them back to work, although we are also aware that employers are, strictly speaking, supposed to be prevented from doing this.[37] This breaks new ground, and raises the question as to whether individual patients should be allowed to follow suit by paying privately to queue jump.

The waiting list problems could be substantially solved by increasing budgets all around. There is talk (as there is in the UK) about the nation not spending enough to provide adequate services for an ageing and middle-class society. But until budgets increase, employers and individual patients are making choices that are threatening the equitable arrangements that have been carefully developed and strengthened over many years. Moreover, the small senior circle of management consultants and health economists advocating competition over the past ten years has commercialised the culture and language, so that policy-makers and providers increasingly think in market terms.[38] The current Minister of Health, for example, wants to move from national to local contracting, in the belief that this will lower costs through competition. If implemented, this policy could backfire, since many providers have monopolies (or could quickly create them).[39,40,41,42,43] The Minister also wants insurers to take over purchasing drugs from manufacturers, without much thought, it seems, to how manufacturers could use divide-and-conquer strategies to increase utilisation and prices.

Implications of the Dutch system for the UK

The need to regulate private health insurance markets

It is instructive that over many years of experience, the Dutch have concluded that private insurance should be either purely supplementary or fully comprehensive (i.e. people would either have public or private insurance and not both), but not in-between. Since the UK does not have, or does not appear to want, a separate and parallel private scheme for more affluent citizens, the relevant part of the Dutch experience for UK policy-makers is the conclusion that private supplemental insurance policies should not duplicate coverage in the public sector and should not compete in an unfair, selective way with the public health care system if equity is to be maintained.

This position would not preclude patients from paying cash for supplementary private services, but it would preclude large national and international health insurance corporations from coming into the UK, under EU rules and recent court decisions, to enlarge and further segment the private UK market by risk.

This position would also imply that the main delivery system (the NHS) should be committed to provide high-quality and comprehensive services to everyone. (It also implies that the main system should be clearer about what services are provided, so that 'supplementary' can be defined and understood by the public.) This is, of course, current UK policy, but not UK reality. The Blair Government also seems committed to such a goal. But Dutch policy is much clearer and more consistent than UK policy about equal access from waiting lists, regardless of how patients' services are paid for. The Dutch would find it unacceptable to give consultants commercial licenses to set up lucrative private businesses while on the public NHS payroll (the infamous 'maximum part-time contract'), or to set up suites of private beds within public hospitals in order to capture some of the profits from these side businesses.[36] Dutch and US experiences indicate that private health insurance should either be made purely supplemental or fully integrated. Simply extending the role of private health insurance and other forms of private financing would threaten the equitable goals of the NHS.

Ireland: trying to make a second tier equitable

Unlike countries such as Canada that have decided to limit private insurance in the public sector to purely supplementary, non-duplicative services, Ireland developed a universal health care system and a private health insurance scheme side by side. Initially, the Irish started a single, non-profit private insurance scheme for the middle and upper classes, a more egalitarian variation of the Dutch approach. But as the universal system has broadened and strengthened, the voluntary policies have largely come to serve as upgrades, by providing more amenities and quicker treatment from the waiting lists. Irish policy-makers have tried to make this second tier equitable, and in recent years they have created one of the most equitable playing fields for competition in health insurance in Europe. Indeed, one might even go as far as to call this approach 'equitable tiering', unless that is an oxymoron. A brief history clarifies the complex issues and values involved.

The development of a mixed public–private system

As in England, medicine was largely private during the 19th century, except for voluntary hospitals, infirmaries at workhouses and a dispensary service established after 1851. Slowly, the Catholic Church and other voluntary associations built and supported a large number of private, non-profit hospitals.[45,46] Before and during World War II, periodic outbreaks of typhus, typhoid, diphtheria and other infectious diseases, as well as tuberculosis, led to intense efforts to detect and control them in a generally impoverished population.[47] There was an alarming rise in venereal disease, particularly among married people, which called for 'more radical measures'. Power over local health measures centralised around the Department of Health, which introduced a bill in 1944 as 'a tidying-up exercise' that added medical inspections of school children, maternal and child care, health and education, and a number of other extensions to the Department's activities. But countervailing powers saw these extensions quite differently.

The Catholic Church held the view, based on the 1931 papal encyclical *Quadragesimo Anno*, that the family (not the State) was the foundation of moral and social order, and that it was a father's responsibility to provide health care to his family. The vigorous new Archbishop of Dublin, Dr McQuaid, reinforced the unpopularity of dispensaries by declaring the public health services to be inefficient, degrading and 'un-Christian'. In response, he strengthened and extended voluntary services provided to the sick and the poor by Catholic and other communal organisations. Dr McQuaid and the bishops formed, along with others, a second proposal: a comprehensive blueprint for re-ordering society so as to avoid state administrative controls and bureaucracies. Doctors were considered allies who would place the public interest above their own. A National Health Insurance Society was proposed, which would control all hospitals and replace dispensaries with health centres, at which all classes would be treated. The plan did not discuss financing, nor how to handle those who did not voluntarily buy policies. Government ministers refused to take it seriously, which confirmed the suspicion that they were arrogant and insensitive. A third proposal came from the Medical Association, which perpetuated the dispensary system for the poor and proposed an insurance scheme for those earning more than 400 punts per year. This preserved private fees and proposed to make them more widely affordable through insurance.

The Government's energetic new chief medical officer undertook a thorough review of the proposals from the Church and the medical profession. He criticised both in detail for covering only the upper half of the population and requiring a means test for public services. Following the influential Beveridge Report in the UK, he and other government leaders proposed that:

- 'free and extended [hospital-based] services should be available to the whole population'

- primary care should be strengthened as the foundation
- the health of families should be promoted, especially through antenatal and maternal health education
- current services should be reorganised at the county and district levels into community-based, integrated systems.

The authors were practising Catholics and did not view their plan as akin to socialised medicine or as contravening Catholic social teachings. In fact, they drew on the ecclesiastical organisation of priests and bishops, and they expected their plan would gain wide public support.

But the Church led public opinion, and objected to what it saw as the State paternalistically taking over the role of family and father, extending its autocratic and bureaucratic control even to instructing mothers and children about how to live their lives. With fresh memories of Nazi power in Italy as well as Germany, the Church hierarchy's reaction was intense. The Department's proposal for a community-based national health service was condemned as 'totalitarian'. Visions of concentration camps and sterilisation were invoked, with socialised medicine seen as suppressing individual liberty. Especially dangerous was the Department's proposal for antenatal and physical health education. Never should the State replace the Church in teaching about sexuality. Senior bishops had strongly reacted to the invention of sanitary tampons as sexually provocative, and the sale of contraceptives had been a criminal act since 1935. They even opposed the Department's plans for controlling the widespread dread of tuberculosis – better done in the Church's opinion by the Catholic-dominated and voluntary Red Cross.

The medical profession was equally adamant, but for quite different reasons. The plan would end their private practice incomes, and the Medical Association joined its self-interest to religious ethics by declaring that state services contravened moral law. They would subvert a father's sacred duty to provide medical care, with the family doctor as his agent, 'restricting clinical freedom or changing methods of remuneration was a limitation on the [divine] rights of the family'. The Church hierarchy responded in turn by echoing the arguments of the medical profession and defending their 'rights'. It opposed any scheme which 'lessened the proper initiative of individuals and associations and the undermining of self-reliance'. In sum, although the Government thought it had the only well-designed plan, backed by years of aggressive and successful campaigns to reduce infectious diseases, its plan faced insurmountable opposition. No party wished to contest the Church on moral issues, so the Church's opposition to a national health care reform on moral grounds ended its prospects.

The ensuing years were filled with struggles over whether medical inspections of school children could be compulsory, whether one-visit dispensary tickets for the poor could be replaced by a medical card for free services, whether committing money from sweepstakes to the hospital building programme was 'an act of piracy' as the consultants claimed in 1950, whether the removal of charges for maternal and child services was 'a Fabian technique', whether the profession was making fortunes out of the misfortunes of the sick, whether the Church hierarchy was sheltered from the harsh realities of Irish life, and so forth.

But no one objected to repairing hospitals and building new ones. The massive postwar building programme added about 7000 beds. Speciality services were greatly improved. Costs grew rapidly, but so did the economy. As these developments occurred during the postwar decades, the Irish Government broadened and deepened its commitment to a public system. It consolidated control by combining 31 health authorities in 1947 into eight regional boards in 1970 with a majority of elected representatives. At the same time, the Government increasingly nationalised financing, making it less local and regressive.[48] The Government saw this as centralising authority by removing power from local boards, which spent health service funds unreliably, and transferring it to more centrally organised services. Health care expenditure rose from 2.5 per cent of gross domestic product (GDP) in 1955 to 2.7 per cent in 1963, but grew to 3.5 per cent by 1968, all of it from increases in hospital-based services.

During the 1950s, the Government came back to its proposals for free, comprehensive services. The medical profession declared they were an 'attack upon the middle classes', took its case to the public and was then joined by the Church hierarchy, which added that expanded services would 'seriously weaken the moral fibre of the people', even though no service would be compulsory under the new proposals. An editor noted 'a striking conformity' between the views of the Church hierarchy and the organised medical profession. In the end, private practice was actually expanded, and the proposal for free child services was reduced from the first 16 years of life to the first six weeks. Nevertheless, the 1953 Health Act established a universal delivery system for people with lower incomes and limited access to public services for the middle classes. The Medical Association came back again in

1951 to its proposal for a voluntary, state-subsidised insurance scheme, which eventually won the day in the creation of the Voluntary Health Insurance (VHI) scheme in 1957, as a mechanism through which people could be more self-reliant and pay for their health care, rather than rely on the State.[49]

During the 1960s, the State continued to press for a free, universal service as the most sensible way forward, and in 1970 an Act was finally passed that effectively brought the dispensary system to an end and created a national health service, 36 years after the Department of Health had first proposed it in the spirit of Beveridge. The share of health care costs from local rates was gradually phased out during the 1970s. The choice-of-doctor scheme, passed in 1972, was considered a landmark of social justice because it replaced the discrimination and stigma of having poor people's doctors with access to any participating doctor. Access for the non-poor to free public hospital beds and to consultant services finally came in 1979 and 1991, respectively. After 1977, the Government also established community care areas and increased community-based services. These developments evolved, one by one, to address issues and needs of the day without national planning. In particular, hospitals were built by a variety of private parties and associations without planning or co-ordination. Costs far exceeded economic growth during the 1960s, increasing from 3.5 per cent of GDP in 1968 to 7.0 per cent in 1979, nearly all of it from hospital-based services.

Meantime, through the 1960s and 1970s, the VHI grew rapidly among the more affluent and expanded its benefits. From the start it was characterised by three principles:

- community-rating
- open enrolment
- lifetime renewability.

It was non-profit and offered the same coverage to everyone, largely focused on quick and superior access to hospital and specialty services. Its handful of policies provided nearly the same coverage, but the better ones offered greater access to the private hospitals and provided extra services. They might be likened to cars, each with all the basics but ever-more amenities from the low-end to the luxury models. The VHI was set up with explicit government control over coverage, benefits and premiums, as almost a second way for revenues to be raised for state-related services.[50]

Initially, VHI looked like the early East-coast Blue Cross and Blue Shield plans in the USA, in that they too offered equitable policies to everyone in the same geographical area on a community-rated basis. But the VHI remained the only source of private health insurance, while competition in the USA led by the 1960s to risk-tiering, exclusion clauses, dropping subscribers once they became seriously ill, and other inequitable practices (*see* Chapter 5).[51] Also, the USA did not continue to broaden and universalise its patchwork of public services and programmes into a national health service. This is the major difference between the USA and both the Netherlands and Ireland. Ireland ended up with a national health service and a widely used voluntary upgrade through a national non-profit insurance scheme that is substantially controlled by the Government as well. One might expect its existence to turn public services into a poor person's service, but the national health services have been steadily upgraded as the foundation of the nation's health service system, alongside the VHI scheme.

Thus, the VHI scheme has developed more equitably than have most private health insurance systems in the world, given that it was a purpose-built second tier. Still, it is considerably more regressive than a system in which funds are raised through income taxes, and the Irish have never developed it into a fully integrated part of the whole, with cross-subsidisation and detailed attention to boundary issues, as the Dutch have done with their upper private insurance tier. About 36 per cent of the Irish population now hold VHI policies, obtained through their employers or through individual subscriptions, and insurance premiums account for about 10 per cent of health care expenditures.[52] Another 15 per cent of expenditure comes from cash payments by patients to pay for the deductibles, user charges and uncovered services in VHI policies, plus cash paid by those who choose not to take out a policy.[53] The other three-quarters of expenditure is accounted for by the Irish national health service.

As the public system in Ireland has become more universal, however, it finds itself in the awkward position of depending on and substantially subsidising the private tier in several ways. It takes care of any problems the VHI policies do not cover. A tax deduction for premiums subsidises VHI and the private hospitals, and within the public hospitals, the private beds, major equipment and separate queuing arrangements are partially subsidised by taxes. Most of the doctors and nurses doing private work have been trained at public expense, with their salary, vacations and pensions paid for by the public system. Contradictions, such as removing the stigma of dispensary doctors, yet solidifying the two-tier access to specialists, or having privileged access subsidised by general taxes, remain unchallenged paradoxes of policy that would generate intense debate about values and priorities in other countries, such as the Netherlands. It leaves the Irish national health service feeling as though it were an inferior service for anyone below middle class who has no private insurance upgrade. By contrast, the UK health system eliminated most two-tier access when it established the NHS, though it allowed (and still supports in several ways) private practice as a way for people to get prompter but unhurried and solicitous service.[54,55,56] To what extent do public funds subsidise private care and to what extent should they? How do the goals of health gain and social gain square with a growing private sector focused on acute intervention after people develop a health problem?

In the late 1980s, a Commission on Health Funding reviewed basic organisational and funding issues, setting the agenda for recent times.[57] While the Commission noted that most countries rely on mixtures of general taxation, social health insurance and private pay or private insurance, it favoured public funding for all health care and gave four reasons:

- it enables a comprehensive and integrated service to develop better than private funding
- it enables transfers from institutions to community care more easily
- contributions better reflect the ability to pay
- equity of access can be assured more effectively.

As for social insurance, the Commission came to the accurate conclusion that it was essentially another form of taxation, but more regressive and therefore less desirable. The Commission felt that access to needed treatment should be available to all, though people above an income floor should pay for general practice – a view heard in New Zealand and elsewhere. Private insurance should be voluntary and supplementary, and the tax subsidy for premiums should end. Ironically, soon after the Commission reached its conclusions, the contradictions of private care were intensified when BUPA built a for-profit, state-of-the-art clinic for complex surgery in 1986, with consultants holding half the equity so that their clinical decisions directly affected both their fees and their return on investment. Citizens and patients do not know about, or understand how, such financial incentives can affect clinical decisions by the specialists in whose hands they have put themselves. Research has consistently found that specialists with a stake in a facility recommend the kinds of services it provides more often, and refer patients to their facility more often, than do specialists without a stake who are treating patients with the same diagnosis.[58] Unnecessary procedures and iatrogenic (medically induced) complications tend to accompany such conflict-of-interest arrangements.

Competition threatens precarious relationships

While the Irish continued to deliberate about the intertwined relationships between their national health service and private up-grade health insurance, the EU was deliberating about the role of competition in historically protected markets. In a series of Directives between 1992 and 1994, the EU required that any non-life insurance company authorised to do business in one EU member state must be allowed to transact the same classes of business in any other state.[59] This means that any insurance company must be allowed to compete in any (or all) EU countries. Self-protective barriers must come down.

The EU Directives challenged the legally protected monopoly that the VHI had as a creation of government. In response to the Directives, the Irish legislature set out to design fair rules for a fair market and created the Health Insurance Act of 1994. The Act 'enshrines in law the three key principles that have formed the basis on which private health insurance has operated in Ireland'.[60] The Act specifies coverages, procedures for registering new policies for approval and many other details. It also permits, if the Minister of Health deems it necessary, a Risk Equalisation Scheme to re-level the playing field between insurers. Otherwise, even with community-rating, 'each insurer would have a strong incentive to 'cherry pick' low-risk lives in order to charge a lower community rate premium or take a higher profit'.[61]

Behind this statement is a more basic point often not appreciated. Competition only benefits society if it rewards efficiency, greater value, innovation and meeting needs. Competition will tend to reward such behaviours only if it meets certain criteria, as listed in Table 6.1: as column 2 indicates, health care often does not satisfy these conditions and has long been regarded by distinguished economists as an area of inherent market failure.[62,63]

When markets are not fair, they reward exploitation of consumers, substitution of inferior services for good ones, selection of low risks, and techniques for minimising payments – all quite easy ways to maximise profits.[64,65] Hence, 'efficient insurers might be driven out of the market by inefficient insurers who are successful in cream skimming … so there is no social gain … [but] only social welfare loss'.[66] Unfair markets also reward collusion, price-fixing,

Table 6.1 Conditions for beneficial competition vs Conditions in health care

1. Many buyers and sellers	1. Few buyers and/or sellers
2. No relation to each other	2. Close, long ties
3. Can purchase from full array of providers	3. Often only a selected array
4. No barriers to enter or exit	4. Very high barriers to entry and exit
5. Full information on prices, quality, services	5. Partial, incomplete, untrustworthy data
6. Information is free	6. Information costly
7. Buyers seek greatest gain/best deal they can	7. Buyers often don't seek much, etc.
8. Market signals quick; markets clear quickly	8. Market signals & market change slow, muddled
9. Price conveys all buyers need to know	9. Price conveys little that buyers need to know
10. No externalities. Buyers experience consequences of their choices fully	10. Extensive externalities, often by construction

withholding market information, private pricing, cornering resources, creating market niches, and other techniques for raising charges and keeping buyers in the dark.[67,68] In these ways, unfair competition can make society and individuals worse off. Even when fair, competition must increase value and efficiency more than enough to compensate for the new costs it incurs. These include the need to gather and quickly disseminate good market information on quality, prices and value, establish market structures, recruit more sophisticated and better paid managers, negotiate and monitor contracts, advertise and market, and make a profit. Often, competition achieves enough new value to compensate for these costs, but given the inherent obstacles to competition in health care markets, it may not. For example, the UK Government transformed the NHS from an administered service to a set of interlocking markets between purchaser and providers, because it believed that competition would increase efficiency; but it gradually abandoned competition because of its financial and political costs, and replaced it with policies of co-operation, though within a framework of separate purchasers.[69] This reflects a realisation that strong purchasing can reap most of the benefits of competition in health care without its substantial costs and liabilities.[70]

The Health Insurance Act of 1994 was a first step in damage control by large corporate competitors selling complicated products (health insurance policies) to innocent and usually uninformed consumers (employers and individuals). To back it up, the Risk Equalisation Scheme designed by the Irish aims to redress imbalances in risk and claims profiles of insurers without dampening their efforts at cost containment and without making any insurer have to share profits earned through greater efficiency and cost control.[71] That is, 'equalisation' should not inadvertently make effective competitors give over some of their profits to ineffective ones. Or, to put it another way, the scheme should redress only financial losses due to higher-risk profiles. This dual goal is difficult to achieve and, in any event, occurs at least a year after a fiscal year comes to a close.[72] Aside from private insurance, some risk-equalising mechanisms such as this may be needed in the UK as 500 primary care purchasing groups or trusts, with very different risk and practice profiles, come on-line.

One notable anomaly in the Irish effort to create a level playing field for competition in health care are the very long waiting periods in the Act before medical services are reimbursed for pre-existing conditions. They are five years for subscribers under 55, seven years for those aged 55–59, and ten years for those 60–64. Such lengths are not empirically or morally justified as protections for insurers against adverse selection by subscribers at risk. They look like a self-serving measure by insurers to get out of covering important risks that lie at the centre of 21st century health care. They constitute legislated discrimination against people with disabilities, chronic conditions, or high risks in the form of 'bad genes'. The chief legitimate purpose for waiting periods is to protect insurance companies from being exploited, for example by someone becoming pregnant or getting cancer and then signing up for a policy. A waiting period of nine months is all the protection a health insurance company needs. Any longer time is pure discrimination against those with on-going health problems who need treatment.

A good deal of mischief is also possible around the meaning of 'pre-existing' and 'condition'. For example, if a woman aged 40 subscribes in January and is diagnosed with breast cancer in March, the medical director of the insurance company may reasonably conclude that the cancer started back in December, if not earlier, and therefore no payments will be made for any procedures during the entire course of the cancer. Such decisions are made by health insurance companies in the USA. With gene profiling, the director might even argue that the 'condition' had begun at conception, 41 years earlier.

Long waiting periods serve only one purpose: to protect the insurance companies from having to pay claims on a substantial and growing set of serious conditions so that they can sell cheaper policies to healthier subscribers. Long waiting periods also shift very heavy and regressive medical costs to those who have known risks, 'conditions' and illnesses. They undermine the Irish efforts to create a second tier that is egalitarian, not only among insurers but among subscribers. Of course, an egalitarian second tier is neither so just nor so cost-effective as having a superior national health service in the first place. Private patients often overpay and do not get good value, because pricing is covert and quality not monitored. Further, two-tier health care increasingly gets in the way of creating integrated services for the major disorders of the 21st century.

To summarise, the 1994 Act attempted to construct a level playing field for fair competition in health insurance, though the very rules of fairness make the Irish market less attractive to outside competitors than markets that allow forms of risk selection. The resulting competition might increase efficiency and contain costs, or it might not.[73]

BUPA challenges the fair market

Soon after this level playing field was set up, an event occurred that is instructive for UK and international policy-makers. BUPA, a major UK health insurance organisation, entered the market and launched the first competitive policies.[74] It posed a serious challenge because it was larger than VHI and had far greater reserves with which to endure an entrenched battle for market share or dominance. Moreover, any new competitor has the natural advantage of not having accumulated a number of subscribers who become seriously ill over the years. In addition, many VHI policyholders were unhappy and ready to change insurers. VHI had dropped coverage for outpatient drugs in 1989, increased out-of-pocket expenditures in a number of ways, and increased premiums for several years.

BUPA's policies imitated VHI's policies in many ways. But BUPA found a loophole in the 1994 Act, allowing it to risk-rate by charging less to younger subscribers and more to older subscribers. This accelerated its ability to draw away older patients and drive VHI into bankruptcy. Since VHI returned almost all its premiums in paid medical services and spent much less on administration than BUPA, it looked as if competition would allow the inefficient to drive out the efficient.[75]

The BUPA challenge to community-rated private health insurance stirred up a storm. BUPA claimed that because the age-graded parts of its policies were not for health care but for cash benefits and other features, its policies were legal.

Indeed, this legal opinion might have been right. It certainly raised a larger issue, namely that the level playing field attempted by the 1994 Act did not apply to cash plans nor to the general private market, where customers also need markets that provide good information on performance, comparative value and quality. Instead, the closed world of specialty private practice makes it impossible for a patient (consumer) to compare prices or information on quality or performance between one consultant and another. BUPA's policies also did not risk-rate nearly so much, or in as many ways, as the health insurance policies that it routinely sells to people in the UK. Their Irish policies were much more equitable than those they are permitted to sell in the UK. But to the Irish, the risk-rating and cherry-picking allowed in the UK was not the issue; the public debate quickly focused on what kind of private insurance market Irish social values would allow.

It was clear from other markets that once risk- or experience-rating begins, it breaks down a community-rated pool like the VHI pool into risk groups or segments.[76,77] We have already described the 'premium death spiral' that occurred in the Netherlands. As the lower risk policyholders are drawn away by cheaper policies, the higher risks are left behind in the community-rated pool, which raises its average costs, further widening the gap between the costs of the risk-rated policies and those of the pool. The spiral accelerates until the community-rated insurer must risk-rate too or go bankrupt. This danger, and the way in which it would force older subscribers to fall back on the public system and thus raise taxes, was quickly highlighted by Irish commentators.[78] Values of family, community and solidarity were invoked. Moreover, worrisome language was found in the core coverage of BUPA's policies. For example, the excluded pre-existing conditions were defined as 'any disease, illness or injury which began before the person … started … membership'.[79] This definition could potentially be used to exclude payment for services even for new or subsequent conditions that had started earlier, even before birth. The BUPA core coverage also stated that benefits would be paid only in relation to diagnoses and treatments accepted by medical standards 'as well as to all the circumstances relevant to the person', a phrase so open to interpretation that it might be used to deny payments for many other possible reasons. The question arose as to why BUPA's officers would choose terms that could so easily be used not to pay for needed services by sick patients unless that was, indeed, their intention.

Meanwhile, thousands of people expressed interest in buying the new policies, and they went on sale, on schedule. The Consumers' Association, the Patients'

Association, and of course VHI pressured the Minister for Health and Children to ban the policies.[80] The Press played a key role by exposing new facts or allegations. Knowing how much further risk selection against the ill could go in the hands of seasoned underwriters, especially with the long waiting periods for pre-existing conditions written into the 1994 Act, a US commentator wrote that some loopholes in the Act were so wide that one could 'drive a herd of Texas long-horns' through it.[81] This echoed the Irish saying one can 'drive a coach-and-four' through something, and journalists delighted in pressing the Health Minister with questions about how easy it would be for BUPA to drive a herd of Texas long-horns through loopholes in the Act. After one such press conference, the Minister announced the withdrawal of BUPA's age-rated policies from the market and said he would establish a commission to review the regulatory framework for fair markets in health insurance.[82] Because of the BUPA challenge, 'the VHI has been forced to redefine its objectives in order to meet the new challenges … [and put] a stronger emphasis on innovative approaches to product design and delivery'.[83] BUPA also regrouped, came out with a new set of acceptable policies, and is actively seeking greater market share using the natural advantages of a new entrant into the health insurance market.

Reinforcing a fair market

The steps taken to make Ireland's health insurance market fairer that followed from the BUPA challenge contain important new policies that any nation should consider in thinking about fair competition in health insurance.[84] First, the Advisory Group on the Risk Equalisation Scheme concluded that the 'single rate community rating' (SRCR) approach in Ireland was not a good system, and, were it not already in place, it should not be used. The most obvious problem of a SRCR is that a single rate for all ages will always be relatively high for young people, whose incomes are usually modest and health needs low – a double incentive not to subscribe. Yet getting the young to sign up is critical to having a balanced community-rated pool of low- and medium-risk subscribers to subsidise high-risk subscribers. In turn, they will be subsidised years later as their risks increase.

The Advisory Group did not even consider as an option the system of extensive risk selection found in the UK market for private health insurance. By contrast, they concluded, the ideal would be Funded Lifetime Community-Rating, namely, a system where premiums would be set according to the age at which people entered, and would be invested to fund future medical costs as subscribers' risks rose with age. To institute this now, however, would have been impractical for several reasons. Everyone currently insured in Ireland is paying the same rates, and these barely cover medical costs plus administrative overheads. How could one switch to an age-of-entry lifetime rate calculated to build up reserves by age cohort, either on top of or alongside the current premium structure and costs that have to be covered each month of the year? What age of entry would be used? The long-term contributors had already paid years of premiums and had the highest costs as a group but with no reserves, because that was not the basis on which they were charged. The Advisory Group, therefore, recommended the next best alternative, Unfunded Lifetime Community-Rating, in which each person's lifetime premium is set according to the age at which they begin to subscribe. If they drop out and re-enter later, they pay the higher rate according to the age at which they re-enter. This scheme provides incentives for young adults to sign up early, so their lifetime rate will be low and not rise in real terms, except as necessary to reflect the general rise in medical costs. Unfunded Lifetime Community-Rating was also the principal conclusion of the Australian Commission that deliberated about fair markets in private health insurance and influenced the Irish Advisory Board.[85]

Second, the Advisory Group recommended that 'the State's responsibility for assessing the competence of consultants for appointment in public hospitals should be extended to assessing the competence of any consultant to practice in the State'. In so doing, the Advisory Group was recognising private practice and its interdependent relationship with private insurance as part of the Irish health care system and not as a separate activity. It is perhaps surprising that the Advisory Group did not apply the same argument to standards and quality for private hospitals and other private facilities. Private patients do not want to pay extra and then find themselves in an inadequately staffed or maintained facility. There are parallels here with the situation in some private hospitals in the UK, where, as we saw in Chapter 4, some private patients are unwittingly exposed to unnecessary risks.

Third, the Advisory Group reaffirmed that the Risk Equalisation Scheme was necessary, but that equalising claims by age and gender was not enough. The Scheme should equalise claims intensity within age or gender groups and make a number of other adjustments. This is sound advice, because claims intensity can vary greatly within a given age or gender group.

Fourth, the Advisory Group reaffirmed competition between insurers as a public policy, but as secondary to community-rating. To make it the first priority would lead to extensive risk selection and discrimination. However, the Group was silent about the inherent and unnecessary risk-rating built into the long waiting periods during which medical treatments for pre-existing conditions (however defined) are not covered. It urged that full economic costs be reflected in payments, and that payment structures between insurers and providers be made more flexible. It also strongly recommended that the VHI be set up independent of the Government as a normal insurance company – a very significant issue for Ireland, but not for most other countries.

Finally, the Advisory Group recommended the use of diagnostic-related groups (DRGs), quality-adjusted life years (QALYs), clinical protocols, and 'fixed price procedures' to encourage cost containment using rational ways to measure costs and quality, a common recommendation that is ethically more difficult than many realise.[86] As in the Netherlands, oversight of the market will be a dynamic process of redefining and adjudicating on market boundaries. Other countries can learn much from the legal and institutional frameworks developed by the Irish about how to make health insurance markets more fair and reward value for money rather than risk selection, de-selection and cost-shifting. Nevertheless, the very existence of the second tier undermines the fairness of the health care system seen as a whole.

Design flaws in having a second tier

The Irish legal framework sets firm limits on unfair discrimination, which are in contrast with what the UK continues to allow in private health insurance, namely:

- community-rated premiums *versus* higher tariffs for older and sicker people
- guaranteed renewal *versus* dropping patients as they get sicker
- open enrolment *versus* insurers choosing whom to cover
- standardised coverage terms *versus* each insurer covering what it likes and how, leaving the rest to the public sector.

Nevertheless, problems remain in the Irish design of its public–private relations. First, although coverage is more standardised in the two sectors, whatever coverage is chosen constitutes two-tier access to those services. Second, as private health insurance spreads, the moral and financial support for good access in the publicly financed health service can weaken. As so many people have quick access by paying for private health insurance, pressure to improve or maintain prompt access in the public system is weakened. For example, at the end of 1997, the Irish Department of Health reported that 76 per cent of adult patients waiting for publicly financed cardiac surgery had to wait more than 12 months.[87] Since the middle classes have quick access to surgery via private insurance, this level of under-provision constitutes pure discrimination against people on lower incomes, similar to the situation in the UK. The quality of facilities and equipment are also different and likely to remain so.

Second, in the Irish case, the premiums are tax deductible, which constitutes a large public subsidy for quicker access and better care for the middle and upper classes. Tax deductibility also makes premiums relatively more costly to the young and those on low incomes, and cheaper to the middle-aged and more affluent who pay taxes at higher rates.

Third, people over 65 cannot sign up for private health insurance, and older people already in the system find the premiums increasingly unaffordable and drop out. Age discrimination is far worse in UK private health insurance, but it is clearly present in the Irish private market as well.

Fourth, the very long and unwarranted waiting periods for pre-existing disorders may keep premiums down, but at a high price for those with chronic problems and disabilities.

Could the UK, or any country, solve these problems, if it started with a clean slate? All except one are solvable. With a funded or unfunded 'lifetime community-rating' scheme, but without a tax deduction, problems two and three could be eliminated. Waiting periods could be limited to (say) nine months, thereby getting rid of problem four. But in the end there is no way around the first problem of inequitable access as long as private insurance coverage is permitted for services included in the public system. In fact, the better the second tier is designed, the more two-tier access and quality will be built into a system. In addition, a two-tier system does not save people money – quite the contrary. Most private insurance has much higher administrative costs, plus profits and marketing, and most private practice is based on non-posted fees so that no viable market actually exists, as it does for hotels or cars. Consequently, the fees charged are exceptionally high. Patients cannot shop for quality and price in the way they can for a good hotel room or a good dinner. Nor are there professional reviewers, as in all good markets, comparing how Mr Jones 'does' hips compared to Mr Scott. In summary, there will always be some private care bought by patients for various personal reasons, but if the private second tier is of any size, those paying the premiums and fees out of their pockets would get much better value if their hard-earned money went to strengthening the main health care system for themselves and everyone else.

Based on the Irish and Dutch experiences, it would seem that using private medical insurance for social purposes in an equitable way requires constant, detailed governmental monitoring and regulation. There is the constant risk of adverse selection and a 'death spiral' or 'race to the bottom' among competing firms. Experience indicates that private medical insurance cannot co-exist fairly with the public system unless it is either purely supplementary with no double coverage for topping up, or a fully comprehensive alternative to the public system. The latter approach can weaken the support for the public system and lead to its decline. This is a basic policy decision that UK leaders need to make, especially in the light of EU rules about markets in health insurance and health care services being open to anyone. Despite these problems (or because of them), both Ireland and the Netherlands have developed specific policies for private health insurance and health care that are notably more equitable than in the UK. Policies that UK leaders need to consider include limits on risk selection, waiting periods and other techniques of risk-rating; guaranteed renewal of one's policy; lifetime community-rating based on age of entry; open enrolment; and consumer-friendly reports on quality and prices.

This central problem concerning equity has important implications for the UK health care debate about private health care. One option is to pursue the same objectives as the Dutch, albeit within different structures, and to maximise equality of access, regardless of the method of payment. This might have a downside in terms of equity of financing, but as a nation the UK might decide that it gave greater weight to equity of access than financing. Another option is to take the best of the Irish system, explicitly accept a measure of two-tierism, and develop rules for financing and provision accordingly. Of course, this raises a pointed question for UK policy-makers – how fair, or unfair, do they think the health care system should be? Whatever they decide, how would the health care system be regulated to ensure that the desired equity goals are achieved? The Labour Government has shown that it is willing to think about equity, but has not yet developed detailed policies on financing, provision or regulation. We have already discussed UK financing and provision in Chapters 2 to 4, and now turn to the regulation of UK health care itself.

References

1   Schut F T. *Competition in the Dutch Health Care Sector*. Rotterdam: Proefschrift, Eramus Universiteit, 1995.

2   Tiddens H A, Heesters J P, van de Zande J M. Netherlands. In: Raffel M W, editor. *Comparative Health Systems*. University Park, PA: Pennsylvania State University Press, 1984: 371–418.

5   Maarse J A M. Netherlands. In: Raffel M W, editor. *Health Care and Reform in Industrialized Countries*. University Park, PA: Pennsylvania State University Press, 1997: 135–62.

4   www.vectis.nl

5   Schut F T. *Competition in the Dutch Health Care Sector*. Ch. 2. Rotterdam: Proefschrift, Eramus Universiteit, 1995.

6   Okma K G H. *Health Care, Health Policies and Health Care Reforms in the Netherlands*. Copenhagen: WHO-Europe, 2000.

7   Schut F. Personal communication (memorandum to authors). 23 January 2000.

8   Light D W. The practice and ethics of risk-rated health insurance. *JAMA* 1992; 267: 2503–8.

9   Maarse H, de Roo A. *Creeping Privatisation in Dutch Health Care*. University of Maastricht: typed.

10 Galbraith J K. *American Capitalism: the problem of countervailing power*. Boston: Houghton Mifflin, 1956.

11 Light D W. Homo economicus: escaping the traps of managed competition. *Eur J Public Health* 1995; 5: 145–54.

12 Schut F T. *Competition in the Dutch Health Care Sector*. Rotterdam: Proefschrift, Erasmus Universiteit, 1995: 132.

13 Light D W, Schuller A S, editors. *Political Values and Health Care: the German experience*. Part I. Cambridge, Mass: MIT Press, 1986.

14 Schut F T. *Competition in the Dutch Health Care Sector*. Ch. 4. Rotterdam: Proefschrift, Erasmus Universiteit, 1995.

15 Schut F T. *Competition in the Dutch Health Care Sector*. Rotterdam: Proefschrift, Erasmus Universiteit, 1995: 134.

16 Light D W. The practice and ethics of risk-rated health insurance. *JAMA* 1992; 267: 2503–8.

17 Schut F T. *Competition in the Dutch Health Care Sector*. Rotterdam: Proefschrift, Erasmus Universiteit, 1995: 141–3.

18 Light D W. The practice and ethics of risk-rated health insurance. *JAMA* 1992; 267: 2503–8.

19 Schut F T. *Competition in the Dutch Health Care Sector*. Rotterdam: Proefschrift, Erasmus Universiteit, 1995: 143.

20 Schut F T. *Competition in the Dutch Health Care Sector*. Ch. 4. Rotterdam: Proefschrift, Erasmus Universiteit, 1995.

21 Schut F T. *Competition in the Dutch Health Care Sector*. Rotterdam: Proefschrift, Erasmus Universiteit, 1995: 143–144, 154.

22 Okma K G H. *Studies on Dutch Health Politics, Policies and Law*. Ch. 5. PhD thesis. Utrecht: University of Utrecht, Faculty of Medicine, 1997: 106.

23 Ibid.: 106.

24 Enthoven A C. *Theory and Practice of Managed Competition in Health Care Finance*. Amsterdam: Elsevier, 1988.

25 Light D W. Homo economicus: escaping the traps of managed competition. *Eur J Public Health* 1995; 5: 145–54.

26 Light D W. The practice and ethics of risk-rated health insurance. *JAMA* 1992; 267: 2503–8.

27 Ibid.

28 Schut F T. *Competition in the Dutch Health Care Sector*. Rotterdam: Proefschrift, Eramus Universiteit, 1995.

29 Advisory Group on the Risk Equalisation Scheme. *Report of the Advisory Group on the Risk Equalisation Scheme: the Minister for Health and Children's independent review of the Risk Equalisation Scheme*. Dublin: Ministry for Health and Children, 1998.

30 Industry Commission of the Commonwealth of Australia. *Private Health Insurance*. Report No. 57. Canberra: Productivity Commission, 1997.

31 Maarse H, de Roo A. *Creeping Privatisation in Dutch Health Care*. University of Maastricht: typed, 2000.

32 Light D W. Managed competition, governmentality and institutional response in the United Kingdom. *Social Science & Medicine* 2001; 52: 1167–81.

33 Light D, Dixon M. A new way through. *Health Serv J* 2000; 110 (5717): 24–5.

34 Lieverdink H. The marginal sucess of regulated competition policy in the Netherlands. *Social Science & Medicine* 2001; 52: 1183–94.

35 Ibid.

36 Maarse H, de Roo A. *Creeping Privatisation in Dutch Health Care*. University of Maastricht: typed, 2000.

37 van Doorslaer E, Brouwer X. Waiting lists in the Netherlands: workers first? *Journal of Health Services Research and Policy* 2000; 5: 129–30.

38 Lieverdink H. The marginal sucess of regulated competition policy in the Netherlands. *Social Science & Medicine* 2001; 52: 1183–94.

39 Marmor T R, Maynard A. Rhetoric and reality in the intellectual jet stream: the export to Britain from America of questionable ideas. *J Health Politics, Policy and Law* 1991; 16: 807–16.

40 Glaser W A. The competition vogue and its outcomes. *Lancet* 1993; 341: 805–12.

41 Light D W. Escaping the traps of postwar western medicine. *Eur J Public Health* 1994; 3: 281–9

42 Light D W. Homo economics: escaping the traps of managed competition. *Eur J Public Health* 1995; 5: 145–54.

43 Marmor T R. Global health policy: misleading mythology or learning opportunity. In: Altenstetter C, Bjorkman J W, editors. *Health Policy Reform: national variations and globalization*. New York: St Martin's Press, 1997: 348–64.

44 Light D W. The real ethics of rationing. *BMJ* 1997; 310: 112–15.

45 Curry J. *Irish Social Services*. 3rd ed. Dublin: Institute of Public Administration, 1998: 112–42.

46   Tormey W P. Two-speed public and private medical practice in the Republic of Ireland. *Administration* 1993; 40: 371–81.

47   Barrington R. *Health, Medicine & Politics in Ireland 1900–1970.* Ch. 7–10. Dublin: Institute of Public Administration, 1987. The following account and details are selectively based on Barrington.

48   Curry J. *Irish Social Services.* 3rd ed. Dublin: Institute of Public Administration, 1998.

49   Byrne A L. *The Voluntary Health Insurance Board: prospects for survival in a competitive environment.* Ch. 3. Dublin: Dissertation in the Department of Social Policy and Social Work, National University of Ireland, University College, 1995.

50   Ibid.

51   Light D W. The practice and ethics of risk-rated health insurance. *JAMA* 1992; 267: 2503–8.

52   Advisory Group on the Risk Equalisation Scheme. *Report of the Advisory Group on the Risk Equalisation Scheme: the Minister for Health and Children's independent review of the Risk Equalisation Scheme.* Dublin: Ministry for Health and Children, 1998: 12.

53   Wiley M. The public/private mix within the Irish medical care system. In: *The Irish Health System in the 21st Century.* Leahy A L, Wiley M W, editors. Dublin; Oak Tree Press, 1998.

54   Honigsbaum F. *The Division in British Medicine.* London: Kogan Page, 1979.

55   Curry J. *Irish Social Services.* 3rd ed. Dublin: Institute of Public Administration, 1998: 112–42.

56   Light D W. The two-tier syndrome behind waiting lists. *BMJ* 2000; 320: 1349.

57   Curry J. *Irish Social Services.* 3rd ed. Dublin: Institute of Public Administration, 1998.

58   Rodwin M A. *Medicine, Money and Morals.* New York: Oxford University Press, 1993.

59   Light D W. Homo economicus: escaping the traps of managed competition. *Eur J Public Health* 1995; 5: 145–54.

60   Advisory Group on the Risk Equalisation Scheme. *Report of the Advisory Group on the Risk Equalisation Scheme: the Minister for Health and Children's independent review of the Risk Equalisation Scheme.* Dublin: Ministry for Health and Children, 1998: 14.

61   Ibid.: 16.

62   Light D W. Escaping the traps of postwar western medicine. *Eur J Public Health* 1993; 3: 281–9.

63   Light D W. The sociological character of markets in health care. In: Albrecht G L, Fitzpatrick R, Scrimshaw S C, editors. *Handbook of Social Studies in Health and Medicine.* London: Sage, 2000: 394–408.

64   Light D W. Bending the rules. *Health Service J* 1990; 100: 1513–15.

65   Light D W. Escaping the traps of postwar western medicine. *Eur J Public Health* 1993; 3: 281–9.

66   van de Ven, W P M M. Perestrojka in the Dutch health care system. *Eur Economic Rev* 1991; 35: 430–40.

67 Light D W. The practice and ethics of risk-rated health insurance. *JAMA* 1992; 267: 2503–8.

68 Light D W. Escaping the traps of postwar western medicine. *Eur J Public Health* 1993; 3: 281–9.

69 Light D W. From managed competition to managed co-operation: theory and lessons from the British experience. *Milbank Quarterly* 1997; 75: 297–341.

70 Light D W. *Effective Commissioning.* London: Office of Health Economics, 1998.

71 *Risk Equalisation and Health Insurance in Ireland: Technical paper on a proposed amended scheme.* January 1999.

72 Byrne A. The voluntary health insurance board: prospects for survival in a competitive environment. *Administration* 1997; 45: 59–79.

73 Light D W. The sociological character of markets in health care. In: Albrecht G L, Fitzpatrick R, Scrimshaw S C, editors. *Handbook of Social Studies in Health and Medicine.* London: Sage, 1999.

74 Seekamp G. BUPA v VHI: How do they compare? *The Sunday Business Post* 1996; 24 November: 32–3.

75 van de Ven's scenario (*see* van de Ven, W P M M. Perestrojka in the Dutch health care system. *Eur Economic Rev* 1991; 35: 430–40).

76 Department of Health. *Draft Regulations Pursuant to the Health Insurance Act 1994.* Dublin: Department of Health, 1995.

77 Byrne A. The voluntary health insurance board: prospects for survival in a competitive environment. *Administration* 1997; 45: 59–79.

78 Fitzgerald G. Proposed BUPA scheme is fatal for our health service. *Irish Times* 1996; 28 December: 12.

79 BUPA Ireland. *Essential Scheme Rules and Table of Benefits.* Dublin: n.d. (Nov 1996).

80 McNally F. Noonan urged to relinquish role as regulator of health insurance. *Irish Times* 1997; 4 January: 1.

81 Light D W. BUPA's Plans to threaten the social basis of health insurance. *Irish Times* 1997; 9 January: 5.

82 Nolan M. Noonan gives BUPA health warning. *Evening Standard* 1997; January 9: 1.

83 Byrne A. The Voluntary Health Insurance Board: prospects for survival in a competitive environment. *Administration* 1997; 45: 60.

84 Advisory Group on the Risk Equalisation Scheme. *Report of the Advisory Group on the Risk Equalisation Scheme: the Minister for Health and Children's independent review of the Risk Equalisation Scheme.* Dublin: Ministry for Health and Children, 1998.

85 Industry Commission of the Commonwealth of Australia. *Private Health Insurance.* Report No. 57. Canberra: Productivity Commission, 1997: 39.

86 For a brilliant new approach, *see* Menzel P, Gold M R, Nord E *et al.* Toward a broader view of values in cost-effectiveness analysis of health. *The Hastings Center Report* 1999; 29: 7–15.

87 Houghton F, Connors T. Private health insurance in Ireland – an issue of particular concern for older people. *Irish Social Worker* 1998; 16: 16–18.

Chapter 7

Regulation for consumer protection

Introduction

Chapters 5 and 6 have shown that governments in other countries with different health systems have always had to take account of private health care financing and provision in their policy-making. In our discussion of the USA in Chapter 5, we highlighted the importance for health policy of establishing firm and detailed rules which reward insurance companies that provide better service and value, rather than reward techniques for minimising payment and coverage. In thinking about possible implications for the UK, we noted the need to create a fair market in which:

- a limited number of comparable policies are sold at open prices and without risk selection
- providers' charges are transparent, so that wholesale and retail buyers (employers, insurers and patients) can shop for price and good value
- insurers and providers are clinically and financially responsible for follow-up care, mishaps and complications surrounding a test or procedure
- insurers and providers offer a package service for a package price, overseen by a regulator with appropriate technical support.

These conclusions were reinforced by our discussion of the Netherlands and the Republic of Ireland in Chapter 6.

In this chapter, we return to the UK, and investigate the extent to which current regulations in the public and private sectors are designed to protect and promote the interests of consumers. The list above focuses largely on protecting consumers *ex ante*, i.e. at the time that they decide which insurer and which level of cover they wish to buy at what price. However, there are other *ex post* aspects of consumer protection that are also covered in this chapter, such as complaints systems when the service of the insurer does not match the expectations of the patient. The chapter shows that there has been a shift towards external regulation of the financing and provision of private health care, together with a move from deterrence to compliance regulation. Nevertheless, the resulting pattern of regulation is still far from optimal, and we propose some further changes.

Health care markets

Standard economic theories of markets start with the assumption that individuals can search for and find a good or service they want. They are able to judge the value of the good or service on offer, and decide whether or not to buy it. For people on reasonable incomes, some health care markets approximate to this ideal. Sticking plasters and cold remedies are widely available at affordable prices and quality is reasonably easy to judge. As long as appropriate regulations for their sale are adhered to, such as the provision of clear information about the dose of a medicine to be taken, then the risks are small.

Other markets for health care goods and services can deviate substantially from the theoretical ideal.[1] In some instances, a good or service will provide no health benefit, or be unsafe, and all consumers will be exposed to clinical and financial risks. Cosmetic surgery[2] and vitamins for general health needs are both examples of goods and services whose effectiveness is arguable. However, more often, the consumer's problem lies in the difficulty of distinguishing doctors or physiotherapists whose practice is unacceptably below standard. Even if they realise this, many consumers of health care will find it difficult to 'shop around' for a service because information on the competence and performance of individual practitioners is often not publicly available.

The complexity of health care also makes it difficult for consumers to know whether a recommended treatment is appropriate for them, or whether the prices quoted in the private market represent good value for money. (Indeed, in some services the full costs are not always apparent at the start of a course of treatment, further increasing the problem.) This can be true for goods and services as diverse as homoeopathy, hearing aids and cosmetic surgery. In short, market mechanisms alone cannot be relied upon to deliver safe, high-quality care to all consumers. Standard regulations for safety and quality need to be established in health care, with credible sanctions against their violation.

These arguments can be put more formally. Economists and sociologists have identified a number of reasons why markets fail, including:

- *Uncertainty*. Needs can be hard to predict and the consumer may not know whether he or she 'needs' medical help until he or she has consulted a doctor. The scope and nature of the service subsequently required can also be hard to predict.

- *Information asymmetries.* Typically, doctors, insurers and other parties have more information about their services and the management of the disease than the average consumer, who will usually know less about insurance or health and health care issues than the professionals.
- *Moral hazard for both insurers and subscribers.* If subscribers know their own health risks (which they tend to do better than most insurers), then they may take out insurance and run up substantial costs for that insurer – moral hazard for the insurer. Conversely, if insurers know subscribers' risks and illnesses, they may refuse to cover part or all of the associated medical costs, raise premiums or refuse to insure them. In the presence of conventional third-party payer insurance, neither patient nor doctor/provider organisation faces any incentives to consider the cost of the treatment selected, since neither bears the cost of the treatment. This can lead to premiums rising faster than prices in other parts of the economy.
- *Adverse selection.* As a result of moral hazard, an insurer may find that it has more higher-risk patients than its competitors, thus driving up the premiums it has to charge its customers. This further discourages healthier patients from taking out its policies, thereby concentrating high-risk patients with that insurer. Eventually, the insurer's financial viability may be threatened.
- *'Cream skimming'.* Insurers and providers can decide not to cover or treat people whose risks and illnesses may cost more than they are paid. As a result, people with high health care needs may fail to get the coverage they need.

Each of these problems might, at least in principle, be addressed separately within the context of a regulated marketplace. For example, where it is found that consumers have poor information about the health benefits of a particular treatment, providers can be required to provide relevant information. It is important to recognise, however, that the theoretical assumptions made generally about the superiority of market mechanisms are not strongly supported in the health care field.[3] This is because, in health care markets, all of the above causes of 'market failure' tend to be present simultaneously, whereas in other markets requiring regulation, problems tend to be less wide-ranging. Thus, for health care markets to work well, it has to be assumed that individuals are the best judges of their own welfare, that they have sufficient information to make sensible decisions, and that their decisions do not significantly affect decisions made by other people. These assumptions are often not met in a number of health care markets in the UK – or anywhere else. Often, the reason why people go to see their GP is precisely because they are not sure what is wrong with them and whether a professional might be able to alleviate the problem. Even when they know, they may find it difficult to decide on the best course of action. In these circumstances, giving them information on the health benefits of a particular treatment may help, but it is unlikely to be enough to circumvent all the problems they face in the health care market.

Regulation is concerned with actions taken by the State to influence the activities of private firms (or of any organised groups of workers such as doctors or commodity traders) in order to protect the interests of those who may be affected by their activities.

The regulation of health care financing

There have been major changes in the regulation of financial products over the last decade. Regulation has been stimulated partly by changes in government policies that have encouraged people to take more responsibility for their own financial affairs,[4] and in part by pensions mis-selling and other scandals.[5] Changes in legislation have focused mainly on life products, such as pensions and life assurance policies, where a purchaser is financially committed to a decision for many years. General insurance products, such as car and private medical insurance, which are typically renewable every year, have received much less attention to date. Yet, as we saw in Chapter 5, there are substantial regulatory issues raised in the USA by practices such as risk-selection, coverage limits and exclusion clauses. Similar practices exist in the UK private insurance market, and this is no surprise since such practices are at the heart of private insurance. This section starts with private medical insurance and continues with other methods of health care financing, including direct payment, since this is becoming more common. It shows that the pattern of regulation of finance and service delivery is complex and hard to justify. Aspects of regulation have recently been strengthened, but it remains unclear how well consumer interests are currently being promoted and protected.

Private medical insurance

Private medical insurance is used to pay for 80 per cent of those treatments that are provided by specialists in private hospitals and clinics, and NHS pay beds. As we saw in Chapter 2, it does not generally cover GP treatments, and only a few primary care treatments. Private medical insurance is regulated as a financial product, rather than as part of a core health service, and regulatory effort to date has focused on organisations that offer private medical insurance products and on the design and sale of these products.

First, companies offering private medical insurance, in common with other insurers, are regulated by the Insurance Directorate, which was formerly based within the Treasury and is now a section of the Financial Services Authority (FSA). The Directorate monitors the financial viability of firms to underwrite insurance, across all kinds of insurance product. The Directorate has the power to withdraw licences, if necessary, and has done so on a handful of occasions in each of the last few years. To date, as we understand it, none of the insurers operating in the private health market has had financial problems warranting action. (As noted in Chapter 2, a number of private medical insurers are owned by very large general insurers. These organisations are financially sound, even if their medical subsidiaries are not profitable.) The Insurance Directorate plays an important role in providing basic assurance about the financial viability of companies.

Second, regulation of the sector is not the task of a single dedicated regulator. This is not an unusual state of affairs – many UK industries do not have dedicated regulators. If there is a risk that a firm in such an industry is becoming too powerful, then the Competition Commission can intervene. This is exactly what happened in the spring of 2000, when BUPA announced that it had bought just over one-quarter of the shares of CHG, the fourth largest hospital group, and had agreed a takeover. The takeover was referred by the Secretary of State for Trade and Industry to the Competition Commission. The Commission is the successor to the Monopolies and Mergers Commission, which investigated the level of consultants' private fees in 1994 (*see* Chapter 4). As its name suggests, its role is to investigate alleged instances of anti-competitive practices, and its remit runs across all industrial and commercial activity. The Secretary of State for Trade and Industry can refer specific companies, or whole industries, to the Competition Commission for investigation. Investigations are undertaken by panels of four to six Commissioners, and reports and recommendations prepared for the Secretary of State.

The Competition Act 1998 strengthened the powers of the Commission, particularly by making its own conclusions more binding on the Secretary of State. Whereas Monopolies and Mergers Commission reports could be disregarded, and the Secretary of State could decide to go against its recommendations, the Competition Act made the Competition Commission the main decision-making body. Under the Act, the Commission has a duty to base its decisions on technical arguments, so that political considerations are marginalised. This has been done partly to offset criticism of some decisions made during the 1990s, which were widely perceived to be politically determined, and not made with the proper interests of consumers or industries to the fore.

In the case of BUPA and CHG, the concern was that the merged group would be too powerful across the private insurance and hospital sectors. BUPA is vertically integrated and has a major presence in both areas. It would have been the largest actor in both sectors, and might have used its market knowledge and power to price services to undermine other firms, or simply to increase consumer prices beyond the levels that would be expected in a more competitive market.

In the course of the investigation, three possible outcomes were evaluated. The first was to allow the merger. The second was to allow the merger on condition that BUPA agreed to separate its insurance and hospital/nursing home businesses. BUPA told the Commission that it would not split itself and would call off the takeover if this was the decision. The third possible outcome was to block the merger and require BUPA to sell its shareholding in CHG. In the end, the Competition Commission recommended that the merger should be blocked. The minister responsible agreed, and the formal announcement was made in December 2000. BUPA then announced that it would sell its shares in CHG.

Thus, the Competition Commission has already exercised its powers in the sector. While the Commission is not an active champion of individual users, it can ensure that consumer interests, in general, are taken into account when firms develop powerful market positions within industries.

Third, the design and selling of private medical insurance products are regulated by the Association of British Insurers (ABI), which is the representative body for general insurance companies, i.e. the industry regulates itself when it comes to policies sold to consumers. Most companies, or at least all the larger ones, but not all that offer medical insurance, are members of the ABI, which has a general Code of Practice for the selling of insurance and a supplementary Code specifically for private medical insurance products. The Code for private medical insurance sets out minimum standards for explaining to customers what is covered and not covered by a particular policy, both in writing and when it is being presented to a potential customer by any salesperson.

Both Codes were developed with member organisations, but the ABI has no formal monitoring system: it assumes compliance. This essentially passive stance, which is analogous to that of self-regulatory bodies for clinicians – which we come to later – does little to promote consumer interests. Rather, it tends to support the interests of insurers, a point underscored by the US experience reported in Chapter 5, and supported by the views of the Office of Fair Trading (OFT) (*see below*). Individual companies may well strive to ensure that the interests of their customers are protected in dealings with hospitals and clinicians – one would expect this in any market. Equally, though, there is little in the Codes to stop companies from doing the bare minimum if they so wish. The new General Insurance Standards Council (GISC), which is in effect taking over the ABI's role, might in time develop stronger codes.

OFT reports

In the early 1990s, a number of problems with private medical insurance became apparent. Prices were rising faster than inflation, and policies were difficult to compare with one another, so that it was difficult to assess the value for money they offered. This came to the attention of the OFT, which is one of the older statutory regulators in the UK, having been created in the late 1950s with a remit to protect the interests of consumers across the spectrum of market activity.

The OFT began with relatively limited powers, and over the years was criticised for being more concerned with encouraging competition than focusing directly on the protection of consumer interests. The OFT's powers have been strengthened, however, particularly by the Competition Act 1998.[6] For example, the OFT now has powers to enter premises and demand documents in the course of its enquiries. If companies are found to be in breach of the Act, the OFT can fine them up to 10 per cent of their UK turnover. The OFT also works with the Competition Commission. (Following the 2001 General Election, the Labour Government announced that it would further strengthen the powers of both regulators.)

Since the OFT has a very broad remit, it monitors developments in a large number of markets, and uses its monitoring information to identify possible breaches of consumer legislation, including the Consumer Credit Act 1974 and the Competition Act 1998. In the mid-1990s, the OFT identified possible problems in the market for private medical insurance and decided to mount an investigation. In its 1996 report, the OFT made a number of criticisms of private medical insurance products, which are paralleled by experiences in the USA (*see* Chapter 5). These criticisms included the following:[7]

- It was difficult for consumers to compare private medical insurance products, and so it was difficult for them to make informed purchases.
- Consumers could find themselves facing sharply increasing year-on-year premiums and were not being properly warned that these rises were likely.
- It was difficult for people being treated to know whether they were being offered the most appropriate treatment, or best value for money. While it is clinicians who decide on treatment, the OFT felt that the insurers could play a more active role in ensuring that patients were informed about their treatment options. The OFT recommended that both the NHS and private medical insurance companies should publicise their protocols on best practices in common formats so that comparisons could readily be made.
- The practice of moratorium underwriting, which typically requires people to declare pre-existing medical conditions and does not allow claims for two years for any problems arising from those conditions, was excessively restricting policyholders' abilities to claim under their policies.

The ABI responded on behalf of the industry in the spring of 1997, promising to review the design of its policies, but also arguing that the OFT's criticism of moratorium underwriting was unduly harsh (though on what grounds it is impossible to determine).

The OFT continued to monitor the industry and, judging that progress was slower than it had expected, published a second report in July 1998. The focus of the second report was on ensuring that proper regulatory controls were in place, with the implication that regulators would be able to ensure that private medical insurance products were properly designed. The Director General of Fair Trading set a deadline of September 1998 for concrete evidence of progress from the industry, and left it in little doubt of his seriousness:

> In this second report, I call for the reserve powers which are to be included in the Financial Services Regulatory Reform Bill … to be employed to regulate moratorium underwritten health insurance. My other recommendations remain, however, directed towards improving self-regulation in this sector. If the health insurance industry wishes to retain a wide measure of self-

regulation, it should, in my view, carefully consider, and then act upon, the recommendations in this report.[8]

The OFT also recommended that:

> *every health insurance policy be accompanied by a clear summary, in standard format, showing what the policy does, and does not, cover … We also recommend that consumers should receive a more comprehensive warning about the likely increase in private medical insurance premiums, supported by reliable data on average increases over the last five years, which we invite ABI to publish.*[9]

The industry responded in September 1998, and promised once again to review the design of policies to meet the OFT's criticisms. It agreed to provide better information about products, including likely rates of increase in premiums, and outlined a strategy based on making the provision of information an integral part of the sales process. It also stated that it had commissioned research to help it develop its longer-term proposals. Following this research, the ABI published new consumer guidance in July 1999, designed to be handed to all potential consumers before purchasing private medical insurance. The guidance explains the main factors that affect the prices of policies, notes the likelihood of premium prices increasing, and the nature of moratorium underwriting. The ABI response was more cautious about the proposals for external regulation of moratorium underwriting. While not saying so explicitly, it was clear that the industry, unsurprisingly, strongly preferred self-regulation to external oversight.

The Director General of Fair Trading had expected that private medical insurance would be regulated along with all other general insurance products by the FSA, under the terms of the Financial Services and Markets Act 2000. This Act had a very difficult passage through both Houses of Parliament, with thousands of amendments being tabled. Early on, it was decided that general insurance products would not be included in the legislation. This seems to have been due to horse-trading over the Bill as a whole.

Thus, general insurance products were excluded from the FSA's remit, with the result that the selling of private medical insurance is still regulated by the industry itself. (However, note that the Insurance Ombudsman Bureau (IOB) is to become part of the FSA's Ombudsman's organisation (*see below*). Selling will remain outside the FSA, but not outside the *ex post* complaints process.)

The OFT has continued to monitor private medical insurance and its associated private medical services. In 1999, it investigated complaints of anti-competitive practices made by private hospital groups, consultants and others against BUPA and PPP Healthcare. The main thrust of their complaints was that both insurers had schemes that favoured some private hospitals over others, and which damaged the commercial viability of those that were not within the BUPA or PPP schemes. The insurers countered that all they were developing were conventional 'preferred provider' arrangements, under which they had identified the hospitals that could offer superior quality of care, better prices, or both. (Indeed, such schemes are, in many ways, desirable for improving value for money for consumers.) The OFT did not publish a full report, but only a press release.[10] This cleared the private medical insurance sector of major competition problems, but once again pointed to the need for insurers to give clearer and more accurate information to policyholders about their rights to treatment.

In July 2000, after further monitoring, the OFT published another press release. On this occasion it was more positive about some aspects of private medical insurance sales:

> *Improved sales literature means that buyers are now better able to compare health insurance products and make an informed choice about them. It shows that after an unwilling start, the industry is beginning to adopt a greater sense of responsibility towards its customers.*[11]

It was not clear how far this statement was based on evidence that consumers could actually compare products in practice. It appears that the OFT was exercising its own judgement and assuming that comparison would be easier based on the existence of new sales literature. This positive statement was tempered by concern at the continuing failure of insurers to publish statistics on the average increases in their private medical insurance premiums over the previous five years, and at the failure to strengthen self-regulation of moratorium-based insurance. The Director General of Fair Trading stated that:

> *Vague warnings about the escalating costs of premiums and the conditions attached to moratorium-based policies do not address all our concerns and we will continue to press the ABI for improvements.*[12]

Four points about the OFT's interest and reports are relevant here. First, the OFT's decision to continue its monitoring of the private medical insurance market is welcome. Without it, the ABI and the industry might not have moved to improve the transparency of insurance policies, even to the extent that they have. Second, the OFT's work highlights the failure of the ABI as a self-regulator with respect to moratorium-based private medical insurance. It is difficult to escape the conclusion that it would not have acted at all without the OFT's presence. The ability of the private medical insurance industry to regulate itself needs to be reviewed as part of a wide-ranging review of the regulation of all forms of payment for private health care, as discussed below.

Third, the reports by the OFT and their subsequent impact highlight both the positive effects that an external regulatory body can have on an industry, and the extent to which an industry can resist proposed changes if it decides to do so. Such resistance echoes the US experience in Chapter 5 and the Irish experience in Chapter 6. The 2000 OFT report shows that consumers have better information about private medical insurance products than they did in 1996. However, it also shows that the industry has not so far satisfied the OFT that it is giving sufficient weight to consumer interests. The US experience over a much longer period suggests ultimately that there are limits to the extent that private medical insurance can be made to work in the interests of the employers and consumers who pay its premiums.

Fourth, the work of the OFT and other bodies representing the public interest needs to be evidence based. A review of the sales literature must be accompanied by research on how the literature is used in practice. Ideally, the OFT should interview a sample of customers to find out what they understand from the literature accompanying policies, and whether in fact customers can assess properly the coverage, risks and values of different policies. Private medical insurers would prefer, if at all possible, to avoid consumers with higher risks. Yet they are the ones who most need insurance. There is little that the OFT or anyone else can do about this in the UK, since the existence of the NHS makes it far easier for insurers to avoid certain risks or certain types of patients. In principle, the NHS covers everyone for acute illnesses. As a result, denials of insurance or selective coverage rarely excite the popular protest that they would attract in other systems.

Strengthening responses to consumer complaints

It is usual to have separate organisations for regulation – rules designed to promote good practices – and for the pursuit of complaints when things go wrong. As indicated above, private medical insurance is regulated as a financial product. Individuals who have complaints have to take them up first with their insurance company. If they are not satisfied, they can go to the Insurance Ombudsman Bureau (IOB).

The IOB was set up by a number of large insurance companies in 1980, as a body for resolving disputes between insurers and individual policyholders. In practice, all firms that offer private medical insurance are members, except the largest, BUPA. The IOB service is paid for by members and is free to policyholders. The IOB runs what is, in effect, an arbitration service between insurer and individual policyholder. The IOB has no legal sanctions, but companies have agreed that its judgements should be binding on them. It is thus a voluntary form of self-regulation. It complements the ABI scheme for the design and sale of private medical insurance, although it covers a narrower range of companies.

The IOB publishes industry-specific information on complaints that it receives. In 1998, 3444 general insurance complaints fell within the IOB's remit.[13] Of these, only 51 complaints (1.5 per cent of the total) were related to medical expenses. This is small in relation to the coverage of private medical insurance policies, which includes over 3 million policyholders covered by IOB firms (see Chapter 2 for data on private medical insurance coverage). These figures might be telling a positive story about the quality of private medical insurance products, but it seems much more likely that the small numbers raise questions about the effectiveness of the complaints system for addressing problems experienced by policyholders.

The Insurance Ombudsman, who runs the IOB, has recognised that there are a number of weaknesses in the scope of the current arrangements for complaints about medical and other insurance, as follows:

- Only individuals can complain, so that employers who provide health insurance for their employees cannot lodge complaints on behalf of people in group schemes.
- The scheme does not cover perceived problems with the coverage of policies, or problems with policies offered by insurance companies that are not members. These restrictions narrow the grounds for complaint to procedural details about the administration of policies.
- The failure of the scheme to deal with disagreements about coverage seems particularly important for private medical insurance, where evidence from overseas strongly suggests that misunderstandings and disputes about what is covered and what is paid are common (see Chapter 5).

The IOB is about to change from being an industry-sponsored regulator to being a government-run regulator as part of the Financial Services Ombudsman's organisation within the FSA. The complexity of the final version of the Financial Services and Markets Act 2000 makes it difficult to be entirely sure how extensive the IOB's powers will be, but they seem likely to include greater powers to pursue complaints with insurers on behalf of individuals. It will be important for the Ombudsman to be widely known and readily accessible to policyholders.

The IOB's remit does not include all private medical insurance companies, because of the legal structure of some insurers. The IOB does not include friendly societies within its scope or other mutual organisations (*see below*). The main gap in IOB private medical insurance oversight is BUPA. It is a member of the Personal Investment Arbitration Service (PIAS) – and thus 40 per cent of private medical insurance policyholders are covered by the PIAS rather than the IOB. This could be confusing to consumers, and the split tends to weaken further oversight of the industry.

The PIAS is run by the Chartered Institute of Arbitrators, originally set up in 1915 to provide a forum for resolving disputes, with the specific aim of avoiding legal actions. Although originally constituted as a private company, the Institute has had charitable status since 1990. It operates over a wide range of industries, including travel and telecommunications, as well as health care. The PIAS is voluntary, and companies choose to join. Figures were not available from the PIAS, but it reported that it 'regularly' had enquiries relating to BUPA insurance and provision. Few enquiries had led to the use of its dispute resolution procedures. However, the PIAS is now part of the new Financial Services Ombudsman's organisation within the FSA. As a result, there is now an opportunity to develop a more coherent complaints system for private health insurance and address the four points listed above. This depends on how well the new arms of the FSA co-ordinate their activities and see themselves as different parts of a single system of regulation.

So what do recent developments in the regulation of private medical insurance amount to? Products and sales remain subject to self-regulation, but company viability and complaints are now under the umbrella of a new statutory external regulator, the FSA. The arrival of the FSA is thus a positive development. However, the FSA does not cover all aspects of private medical insurance, and oversight is fragmented. This reflects the fact that the regulation of private medical insurance has grown up piecemeal, often as a result of wider decisions made about the far larger general insurance market. This complex pattern of regulation seems unlikely to promote consumer interests wholly successfully. The current approach can be improved upon. The goal should be to have a single, visible, and consumer-friendly mechanism for registering complaints and having them addressed in an effective and timely fashion. The new General Insurance Standards Council, which is a new self-regulatory body, might move us towards that goal.

We also note a shift in emphasis from deterrence to compliance regulation. The deterrence model employs *ex post* mechanisms: people are allowed to carry out their business unhindered, but sanctions will apply if they are found to have broken the rules governing their work. Thus, the Insurance Directorate of the FSA does not act until it perceives that an organisation has transgressed, relying on the notion that an investigation is something to be avoided. The avenues for the pursuit of complaints can usefully be conceived as another example of a deterrence mechanism. Compliance, in contrast, involves *ex ante* actions. Individuals or firms are monitored as they carry out their work, and sanctions can be applied if they fail to comply with the relevant rules. Baldwin[14] argues that the compliance approach is more appropriate to the majority of contemporary problems, where the emphasis is on avoiding problems occurring in the first place. In effect, the OFT has moved from being a deterrence-style regulator to a compliance one in the case of private medical insurance. This is the right direction in which to be moving, but it is not reasonable to expect the OFT to devote substantial resources to this policy area indefinitely, given its other responsibilities. Indeed, it is unlikely that the OFT will sustain its current activities in relation to private medical insurance. Thus, we recommend that people who take out private medical insurance should be given their own compliance regulation (*see the end of this chapter*).

The current regulations reflect the underlying values of those who shape them, with those doing the shaping including governments, consumers and the private health sector. In the case of private medical insurance, it is clear that regulation has not been a priority under governments of any persuasion, perhaps because private insurance has been regarded as a small-scale, niche market. This situation may change in the wake of the NHS Plan and the Concordat. Government ministers want a more explicitly mixed economy of health care provision. As a result of such developments, there needs to be a review of existing regulation and complaints arrangements in the private sector. The Labour Government has also been more proactive in promoting the interests of consumers than its predecessor, and this too leads to cautious optimism about further progress in this area in the future. For progress to be made, though, the Government needs to look at private financing overall, and thus we turn to other forms of payment.

Protecting cash customers

Twenty per cent of private hospital treatments are now paid for by individuals, the figure having grown substantially during the 1990s.[15] The clinical and financial risks faced by these individuals will be broadly similar to those experienced by people with private medical insurance. People who experience problems relating to the charges for their treatment can take this up with the hospital. However, if they cannot resolve their problem, the only recourse they have is to civil law.

Some private providers have schemes to help private individuals to pay for their treatment. Nuffield Hospitals, for example, has a scheme called Fixed Price Direct. These schemes offer unsecured loans to help people to spread the costs of treatment over a period, and so are similar in nature to loans for cars and holidays. Again, there is no specific protection available if problems arise, although the schemes are covered by general consumer legislation, which means that the terms of any loan have to be clearly stated to potential customers.

We were not able to determine how well this type of scheme is working, although Nuffield Hospitals stated that it had experienced fewer problems with them than with other forms of payment, and put this down to the transparency of the arrangement for consumers.

Far more problematic than loans is the situation in which patients are required to pay cash in advance of treatment. Cosmetic surgery exemplifies this, as we noted in Chapter 3. Whether using Nuffield Direct or paying a cosmetic surgeon, patients can commit thousands of pounds and thus bear both financial and clinical risks without knowing that their treatment will be successful. There are no comments in the NHS Plan about self-payment.[16] This is a noteworthy gap in the Government's approach to the regulation of health care financing.

We support the views of the Health Committee of the House of Commons that pre-payment for expensive medical treatments should not be allowed.[17] However, the Health Committee did not broaden its arguments and call for fair contracts for individuals or employers wherever any form of self-payment is involved. There would be three key elements to this. First, paying patients should know in advance how much their treatment will cost and what they can expect when things go wrong. Second, all private practitioners should be required to post fixed prices for a full package of procedures and tests, including the costs of any 'hidden extras' and follow-up care for a fixed period (which should be at least 30 or 60 days). The follow-up clause would be similar to any service with a limited warranty, such as car repairs. Third, some insurers and hospital providers, as we noted in Chapter 3, are moving towards explicit pricing of their own accord, so it ought to be possible for all insurers and providers to price whole packages of care.

Health cash plans

As we saw in Chapter 3, about 6 million people contribute to health cash plans for a range of primary care services and also fixed sums for hospital stays. The total amounts spent on health cash plans each year are much smaller than for private medical insurance, at £250 million versus £2 billion for private medical insurance, but the market is growing and new organisations have moved into the market in recent years.

Traditionally, organisations that offer health cash plans have been mutuals, which are 'not-for-profit' organisations, technically owned by their members. Most providers, including larger ones such as Foresters and Benenden Healthcare, are friendly societies, a special class of mutual that is not allowed to offer general insurance. Friendly societies have been regulated since the late 18th century,[18] but there have been important changes in regulation in recent years. The Friendly Societies Act 1992 created the Friendly Societies Commission, whose principal concern was the ability of societies to write policies. It was the body authorised to register and de-register societies. The Friendly Societies Commission will be integrated in the FSA in 2001; this is another element in the move towards more integrated external regulation by the FSA, as already noted above in relation to private medical insurance.

The 1992 Act allowed friendly societies to own, or enter into partnerships with, other kinds of organisation for the first time. Thus, some societies have been able to create subsidiaries that can offer general insurance, as in the case of Manor House Friendly Society, which now offers a private medical insurance product. This is a good example of a development that blurs the boundaries between different financial products, and highlights the need for better integration of regulation for different methods of payment for private health care.

Friendly societies have not hitherto had a formal complaints scheme. Societies themselves tend to the view that mutual status itself is sufficient to assure the proper conduct of business with members. In practice, there are limits to the extent to which mutuals are member-driven. Individual members may well find it difficult to obtain redress for any problems that arise, and so they need access to an independent review body for complaints.

In addition to friendly societies, there are three types of financial services organisation that are not covered by any of the arrangements we have outlined above. First, there is the largest health cash provider, HSA Healthcare. It is a mutual organisation, but not a friendly society, and as a result it is not currently accountable to the Friendly Societies Commission and will not be accountable to the FSA. Its position is broadly analogous to that of BUPA in the private medical insurance market in that, once again, the largest organisation is not regulated to the same extent as other organisations in the same field.

Second, a number of large commercial organisations have moved into the health cash plan market, including Boots, the pharmacy chain and Abbey National. They are subject to general company legislation, and so must comply with consumer protection legislation, which gives consumers basic protections for goods and services provided. They will not, however, be covered by the FSA for the sale of cash plans. Again, this points to the need for review of the regulation of health cash plans, ideally alongside a review of the regulation of private medical insurance.

Third, there are now dental insurance products that have the main features of health cash plans, but for a single service. A good example is the market leader, Denplan, offered by PPP Healthcare. Premiums are of the same order as health cash plans, at £10–£15 per month. Each individual policyholder nominates a dentist, and then makes monthly payments to Denplan, which, in turn, pays the dentist when needed. In return, individuals are entitled to all normal routine dental treatment without charge, plus accident and emergency cover, and a cash lump sum if they have a hospital stay for dental treatment. Denplan is covered by the arrangements that cover PPP Healthcare, including membership of the IOB. For this particular plan, self-regulatory protection and complaints mechanisms are in place.

Summing up

Looking across the financial sector as a whole, the trend in recent years has been to create more integrated regulatory structures that cover many different types of organisation, since any one organisation may now offer several different products. There has also been a shift, albeit incomplete, from *ex post* to *ex ante* models of regulation. The umbrella structure of the new FSA is a product of this thinking. It takes a step in the right direction for regulation of private health care financing, even though it covers only some aspects of financing, excluding self-payment.

It appears that, by oversight rather than design, the financing of private health care remains a partial exception to this general trend towards umbrella, external regulation by statute. The Government needs to develop more integrated regulatory structures. Tables 7.1 and 7.2 summarise the current situation. Table 7.1 shows that assurances about some products have improved over the last four years, mainly because of the creation of the FSA. Nevertheless, there is still a patchwork of regulators. Individual products can be regulated by several bodies, and the regulation of different methods of payment is poorly co-ordinated. Table 7.2 emphasises the point that, while some progress has been made, consumers are still not central to policy thinking

Table 7.1 Changing pattern and nature of regulation of private health care in UK

Aspect of private finance	Identity of regulator and type of regulation, 1998	Identity of regulator and type of regulation, 2002
PMI market/competition	Reports by OFT and Competition Commission. Deterrence regulation.	Continuing interest of OFT and Competition Commission. OFT move towards compliance regulation.
PMI firms' viability	Insurance Directorate. Deterrence regulation.	Insurance Directorate within FSA. Deterrence regulation.
PMI design & sales	Self-regulation by ABI.	Self-regulation by ABI.
PMI complaints about policies/claims	IOB and PIAS.	IOB and PIAS within FSA. External compliance regulation.
Out-of-pocket payment	None	None
Health cash plans	Friendly Societies Commission.*	Friendly Societies Commisssion within FSA.

*Not all health cash providers are friendly societies. HSA is not covered.

Table 7.2 Current oversight of payment for private health care

Method of payment	Assurance that policies are clear and comparable?	External assurance that policies have fair terms?
Private medical insurance	OFT is pressing insurers. Evidence needed that consumers can compare policies. Insurer resistance to some OFT proposals.	Voluntary – self-regulation by ABI. Evidence lacking about fairness of policies.
Friendly societies	None, but may improve under FSA.	None, but may improve under FSA.
Cash payment	Not applicable	None
Health cash plans	None. May improve for people who pay into plans covered by FSA.	None
Dental insurance	Voluntary – self-regulation by ABI.	Voluntary – self-regulation by ABI.

about regulation. The goal should be a one-stop, accessible and consumer-friendly regulator.

Regulation of the provision of private health care

Just as the regulation of financing private health care is undergoing change, so is the regulation of its provision, both at organisational and professional levels. This section discusses the Inquiry into the Regulation of Private and Other Independent Healthcare by the Health Committee in the first half of 1999, since it provides an excellent summary of the weaknesses of regulation up to that time. This is followed by an account of the Government's response over the following months, and a discussion of two key areas – the governance of medical work and the regulation of primary care markets – using dentistry as an example. These key areas are illustrative of wider developments in the regulation of private health care provision.

In order to set the discussion in context, we first describe the accountability arrangements for private hospital care.

Assuring good clinical quality: accountability

The material presented in Chapters 2 to 4 highlighted the fragmented nature of the relationships between private insurers, private hospitals and consultants. If we trace who holds what information, it is easier to understand the structures surrounding private hospital-based treatment, and to analyse the effects of current and proposed regulations. Incomplete information is held by different parties, as follows:

- It is not usual for private providers to have access to NHS patient notes, so relevant information will come only from contact with the patient, and possibly in letters from referring GPs. Different providers thus have different and incomplete information on patients
- Individual insurers have information about the people who insure with them, and who may be treated in many hospitals run by a number of organisations. Any one insurer will be able to see only part of the 'jigsaw' of provision. They will not have information on the 20 per cent of people who are treated without insurance. (Note that it may not be desirable for insurers to have complete information, if it leads to them having undue market power. The goal is therefore to achieve a balance that does not jeopardise the interests of consumers.)
- Insurers have information about individual doctors who treat their insured patients, but they do not share it with one another. If a doctor only does one private session a week, he or she may treat one BUPA patient, two PPP patients, and one each with a policy from WPA, Norwich Union and Prime. Each insurer will therefore know only a little about that doctor's private work that week. This is in contrast to the USA, where insurers do share information (*see* Chapter 5).
- Private hospital groups will have information about which doctors are doing what work on their premises – though only on their premises, so again this may only be a session's worth of work each week.
- Individual insurers and hospital groups only know part of the story of private work, and little or nothing of their doctors' ongoing NHS commitments. Larger organisations, such as BUPA, have the best information, and told us that some consultants do enough work for their insurance side to make accurate assessments of the quality of their work. Even BUPA has a partial view, however, with most consultants earning no more than £10,000 each year from BUPA sources.[19]

The groups that have the best information are the hospital consultants, their Royal Colleges and other specialist organisations. Consultants know what their own work patterns are, and are in a position to pool data from their NHS and private practices to evaluate the quality of their own work in order to identify poor practice and to raise standards overall. To date, however, they have been poor sources of such information. In principle, the best way forward is to require consultants to record and publish their work patterns and data about their clinical performance. Given the Government's intention to make greater use of private hospitals, signalled by the Concordat, this would seem to be the natural next step. Medical power remains a major barrier to progress in this area, but the current debate about improving medical accountability and reporting all adverse incidents may encourage data collection across the public and private sectors (*see below*).

Fairer public–private relations

The current structure of the health sector generates these problems of information fragmentation and weak accountability, particularly relating to the work of consultants. The fragmentation of financing and provision makes it difficult for any one organisation to work out how well consultants, their main contractors, are performing. The division of responsibilities for the financing and delivery of care means that it is unclear who should be held to account when things go wrong, as they are certain to do in health care.

The goal is to measure the quality and outcomes of all clinical services, in order that patient interests can be promoted and protected, whether they are treated in the public or private sectors. This is a proposal for the future. The situation facing the Health Committee when it started its Inquiry into the Regulation of Private and Other Independent Healthcare in 1999 was rather different – there was no NHS Plan, no Concordats, and a Secretary of State for Health who was uncomfortable discussing private hospital care, never mind acting to regulate it.

The situation would be improved if insurance companies were to pool all of their information about doctors, so that there was a single database of all privately insured people who had been treated. This would increase the amount of information about any one doctor, by pooling all cases that the doctor treated. The same would apply to private hospital groups, which could pool their data to increase their knowledge of consultants' work. Indeed, since the hospitals also know about the 20 per cent of people who pay out of their own pockets, their databases would be more complete.

Even better, it should be possible to pool data about a consultant's work in all settings, including the NHS. There are hints that the Government was beginning to think along these lines in the NHS Plan.[20] The Government expects the NHS to move towards greater transparency under the banner of 'clinical governance'. Best of all, the Government could use the Concordat to pool information about the work of consultants. The NHS Plan does not set out specific steps that the NHS should take, but we recommend that trials of information-pooling should go ahead, initially to see if there are significant differences in patterns and standards of work in different settings.

Concerns about quality on behalf of private patients

During the first half of 1999, the Health Committee undertook an Inquiry into the Regulation of Private and Other Independent Healthcare.[21] The Committee questioned a range of witnesses including representatives of private hospital groups, consumer representatives, the Department of Health and the (then) Secretary of State, Frank Dobson. In the course of their questions they ranged over many issues, including perceived shortcomings in the regulation of clinicians working in private settings, whether new NHS bodies such as the Commission for Health Improvement should act as a regulator for private medicine, and the need to develop regulation of both financing and provision at the private health/social care boundary.

The Health Committee chose to focus on a small set of problems that it judged to be important, particularly those arising in elective surgery, cosmetic surgery undertaken in small clinics, and the treatment of people with mental illnesses. It noted that it received little written evidence about complementary therapies, and so did not comment on them. The financing of health care was outside the remit of the Inquiry. The Committee judged that current consumer protections in the services reviewed were inadequate, and made 39 recommendations for changes in the ways in which private health care is managed and regulated.

The key conclusions of the Committee were that:

- There was clear evidence that the market for cosmetic surgery failed to treat some patients honestly and fairly. The Committee proposed a number of changes in the way that this market is promoted and regulated. Their recommendations included tighter rules on advertising, changes in the way that payment is generally made (they judged that pre-payment was unacceptable) and strengthening of professional regulation of this particular branch of surgery. There should also be access to appropriate complaints procedures to ensure that people are better protected than they are at present if their surgery goes wrong.

- There were problems with the co-ordination of NHS and privately provided mental health care. The Committee recommended a number of measures to improve co-ordination, including the NHS taking control of local planning of services. This is a radical proposal, as this could effectively bring the planning of all private mental health care under the control of the NHS.
- There was a lack of clarity about the status of NHS pay beds, which were part of the NHS, but in practice not subject to all of its rules. The Committee recommended that the status of pay-bed services should be clarified by making them subject to the same rules that govern all other NHS services, including clinical governance arrangements.
- There was inadequate accountability of consultants working in private hospitals, whether to the hospitals or any other organisation, for the quality of their clinical work. The Committee recommended that Medical Advisory Committees (or where they did not exist, the hospital chief executive) should oversee clinical standards in each hospital. Thus, they proposed arrangements that would parallel those for clinical governance in the NHS.

The Health Committee has therefore proposed a mixture of strategies in response to the problems it identified, ranging from changes in advertising rules, to clinical governance, to a new regulator. The strategies address three distinct structural issues, namely:

- Problems relating to the *governance of clinical work* in private hospitals and clinics, particularly as they relate to consultants.
- Problems that occur at *boundaries*, covering both the NHS/private health care and private health/social care boundaries.
- Problems in *retail markets*, using the example of cosmetic surgery to illustrate the problems that can occur.

Solutions would have to involve the co-ordination of planning and delivery of services across public–private boundaries. The Committee proposed that:

- There should be an independent regulator for health care outside the NHS (*see* Figure 7.1), accountable to the Government.
- The regulator would focus on the quality of care as well as the appropriateness of premises. It would co-ordinate its work with that of the National Commission for Care Standards, the regulator of social care created by the Labour Government in the Care Standards Act 2000.

Figure 7.1 Proposed structure for regulation of health care outside the NHS*

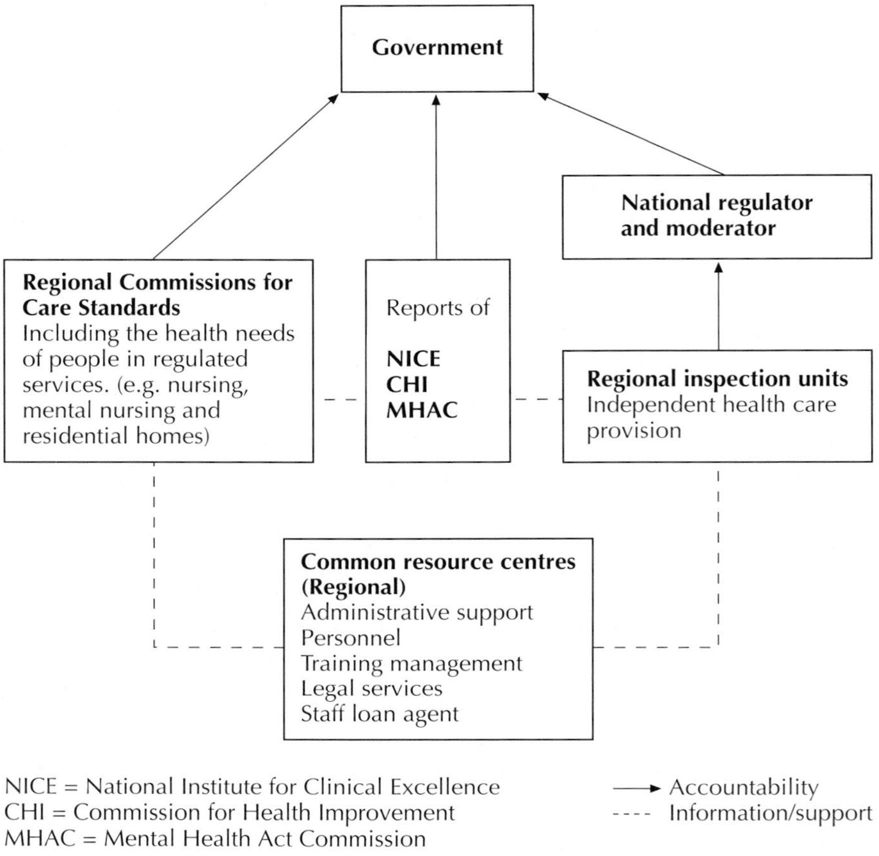

NICE = National Institute for Clinical Excellence   ⟶ Accountability
CHI = Commission for Health Improvement   ---- Information/support
MHAC = Mental Health Act Commission

*Adapted from Health Committee. *The Regulation of Private and Other Independent Healthcare*, 1999: xli.

- There should be a national moderator for private health care, who would be 'required to assess whether emerging techniques and technologies pose any risk to patient safety', and to maintain a list that would be reviewed annually.

Inevitably, in a relatively short inquiry, there were many areas that the Committee did not tackle. There was little mention of the regulation of nursing, or of how the proposals would mesh with the Government's proposals for strengthening the wider regulation of health professionals (*see below*). Interestingly, the Committee did not comment on any of the equity implications of private health care (*see* Chapter 8). The report did, though, summarise a number of important issues relating to consumer protection, and recognised the importance of public–private boundaries in thinking about regulation. It stated in the clearest terms that inaction was no longer an option, because the number and nature of problems were too great to ignore.

Before the Health Committee had published its report, the Government published a consultation document about the regulation of private health care.[22] It acknowledged that the main legislation covering private health care, the 1984 Registered Homes Act, was not working well. The Act had been designed principally with residential and nursing homes in mind, and sought to ensure that minimum standards of accommodation were provided. This approach did not translate well into private health care, where the quality of premises is a poor indicator of the quality of care. Representatives from private hospital groups told us that they saw the Act as an irritant. It was largely irrelevant to them and did not help patients obtain any assurance of good-quality care. It was a regulatory burden that brought no benefits.

The Government also agreed that the introduction of its new policies in social care, designed to strengthen regulation of both domiciliary and nursing home care, meant that it was an appropriate time to review arrangements for the regulation of hospitals and clinics. Yet the consultation document focused mainly on the regulation of premises, continuing the thinking in the 1984 Act. In places, the document admitted that quality of care was an appropriate focus for regulation, but its proposals covered only the physical quality of premises in which the care was provided. The document also proposed that a new regulator should be introduced with powers to stop doctors practising privately if they had been suspended in the NHS for any problem that might compromise patient safety. There were no detailed proposals on the regulation of the boundaries between private health and social care, or issues that directly affect patient care.

During this period, Frank Dobson was still Secretary of State for Health. As already noted in Chapter 4, his preference was to leave the private sector alone. The consultation document suggested that this was still the Government's preference, but that it found itself in a position where it had to act. The need to do something was partly of its own making, as its action to alter the regulation of social care had made the Registered Homes Act 1984 redundant, and action on private health care was one consequence. The Health Committee's work, though, revealed other problems that could not easily be dismissed.

The Care Standards Act 2000

In July 1999, Frank Dobson was succeeded as Secretary of State by Alan Milburn. There were soon signs that the ground was being laid for a change in policy on private health care. Alan Milburn made a speech in December 1999,[23] which indicated that the Government was interested in discussing new types of public–private partnership for the provision of health care. As noted in Chapter 4, this was followed in early 2000 by statements from the Prime Minister and Alan Milburn, stressing their desire to discuss new forms of partnership with private providers.

The Care Standards Bill was published in December 1999. It largely reflected the thinking in the earlier consultation document (*see above*), rather than the new thinking being promulgated by health ministers at the time.[24] As the Bill began its passage through the House of Lords, it became clear that the Government was proposing only mimimal changes to the existing legislation. In contrast to the main part of the Bill, which dealt with the regulation of social services, the clauses relating to private health care proposed continued regulation of premises only.

As the Bill neared the end of its time in the House of Lords, it became apparent that Conservative and Liberal Democrat spokespersons had three main concerns with it:

- The focus of regulation was on premises rather than on services, which they argued would do little to enhance consumer protection. Baroness Nicholson, who had had family experiences of the lack of redress available when problems occurred in private hospitals, was particularly concerned about this aspect of the Bill, although she was not alone.
- The identity and nature of a new regulator for private health care was unclear, and so needed to be thought about more carefully. There was no co-ordination proposed between NHS and private sector regulators. Some speakers called for the newly established Commission for Health Improvement to oversee both NHS and private health care, although this particular proposal was strongly resisted by the Government.
- The scope of regulation was said by critics to be too narrow. It was not clear, for example, that all doctors working in small-scale settings – including private GPs – would be covered. Ministers insisted this was not the case, but this aspect remained a bone of contention.

As a result of Opposition pressure, the Bill was strengthened in relation to consumer protection through the taking of reserve powers by the Secretary of State, i.e. statutory instruments and guidance would be developed after the Bill passed into law. The quality of this guidance will significantly determine the nature and strength of any new measures.

In addition, with regard to the identity of the regulator, the National Care Standards Commission will be responsible for regulation, which offers the possibility of better co-ordination of the regulation of social and private health care in the future. There are also provisions for co-ordination of the work of the National Care Standards Commission and the NHS Commission for Health Improvement, though again the precise form of this relationship remains to be worked out. The National Care Standards Commission starts work in April 2002. The Government is consulting on regulations and minimum standards for private health care.[25] This suggests that there has, finally, been a shift towards regulation of services. The Government has also committed itself to improving the communication of information about hospital doctors subjected to disciplinary procedures in either the NHS or private hospitals, so that all relevant parties are aware that a particular doctor has been suspended.[26]

In summary, the Health Committee's report marked the formal start of serious policy-making for private health care. It prompted the Government into action – and even if its first thoughts lacked some coherence, government thinking has now moved on. The Committee took the protection of consumers as a major theme of its report and made a range of helpful recommendations to this effect. The Committee could have gone further and proposed a framework for protection of consumer interests in all private health care settings, and linked this to a discussion of the equity implications of having a private health care sector in the UK (*see* Chapter 8). But this is to cavil about an important inquiry, which has set out key issues of consumer protection more clearly than any other recent document.

The regulation of doctors: inadequate protection of patients

Whatever the strengths or weaknesses of the Care Standards Act 2000 regulations, the safety and quality of care will crucially depend on the quality of private practitioners. Traditionally, the quality of medical care was largely the province of the individual practitioner. Once trained, they were expected to maintain their skills with little or no oversight or formal requirement to do so.

Over time, the situation has changed, and there are now more formal expectations placed on doctors in respect of in-service training and participation in clinical audit. At their best, these and other quality assurance processes lead to the delivery of high-class services to patients. As in all walks of life, though, the best is not achieved in all places and at all times. In the case of doctors, this fact has been highlighted by recent high-profile cases that have come before the General Medical Council (GMC), such as the cases of GP Harold Shipman and the gynaecologist Rodney Ledward.

The GMC is the self-regulatory body for the medical profession, which was originally set up following the Medical Act 1858, and whose functions are currently defined by statute in the Medical Act 1983. As a regulator, the GMC is responsible for registering doctors and for disciplining them – or in the GMC's own words, 'maintaining good medical practice and preventing and managing poor practice'.[27] These responsibilities apply in all places where doctors work, in both the private sector and the NHS.

Within this broad definition of its role, the GMC's activities tended until recently to focus on administrative abuses and doctors' general behaviour towards patients, rather than clinical work itself. The GMC has not actively monitored doctors – rather, it has been an essentially passive regulator for problems as they arise. (Note that it is not clear whether an appropriate proportion of all complaints find their way to the GMC, or indeed other regulatory bodies.) For cases that it considers within its remit, the GMC undertakes an initial investigation. In the most serious cases, GMC disciplinary procedures can lead to formal hearings, where the ultimate sanction is the removal of a doctor from the Register. The GMC is, therefore, a regulator designed on the deterrence model, and has not hitherto concerned itself with the active monitoring and regulation of doctors' routine activity. Or, put another way, the GMC is simply not designed to be proactive and protect patient or consumer interests.

There has been considerable debate about the role of the GMC, and medical self-regulation in general, in the wake of the high-profile cases involving heart surgeons in Bristol, the gynaecologist Rodney Ledward, and others. Most of the policy proposals, however, have focused on the current state of affairs and on doctors working in the NHS.[28,29] These proposals include the creation of new organisations within the NHS for assessment and retraining of doctors. The GMC is to accredit doctors regularly during the course of their careers. These proposals can be added to wider initiatives, such as the publication of

National Service Frameworks setting out explicit clinical standards for a wide range of services. Doctors will still control most of the review processes. However, the State is taking an ever-more active interest in the quality of those processes, and placing expectations on the medical profession that reviews will be undertaken properly. On balance, therefore, clinical quality is likely to improve in the NHS.

As we have seen in the discussion of the Care Standards Act 2000, it remains to be seen whether equivalent accountability structures are put in place in the next two years for the private sector. The Government appears to hope that the Concordat will lead to NHS standards being applied in private hospital settings, on the basis that private hospitals treating NHS patients should be subject to NHS regulations. It is doubtful, however, that equivalence will be achieved in the private sector – which is why the regulations under the Care Standards Act are so important. It looks as if consumer protection in private hospitals will continue to be weaker than in the NHS in the future. This is not the same as saying that the quality of care will necessarily be poorer, since this depends in part on the quality of the individual doctor, but patient protections will remain weaker.

While it might seem obvious that the next step is to introduce external regulation of doctors, whichever sector they practise in – so that the State regulates them directly rather than licensing the GMC to do so – the political reality makes this difficult. The problem is well captured by Salter:

> *[the State] now knows that reliance on the profession to manage its own process of internal organisational change is gambling against history. On the other hand, the introduction of reform through simple policy fiat, be this clinical governance or some other initiative, is not going to work while an unsympathetic profession controls the power structures necessary for policy implementation. Something more sophisticated is required. The most convenient solution for the State is the manufacture of a new set of power relations within the profession capable of, and committed to, the introduction of comprehensive reforms in the governance machinery ... Self-regulation remains, but in the context of a corporatism that has been significantly rebalanced. To achieve such a realignment within the profession, the State needs not only the artillery of actual, or more probably threatened, legislative intervention in the organisation of medicine but also the massed ranks of public pressure.[30]*

As Salter suggests, a re-balancing of power relations within the medical profession, so that governance mechanisms are reformed, may suit both the Government and medical profession. The Government has indicated that it wants reform of consultants' work (*see* Chapters 4 and 8), which may lead to changes within the NHS. According to Salter's analysis, the Government also needs to step up pressure on the profession to accept closer scrutiny of private work, integrated with NHS scrutiny. This is, after all, the logic of the Concordat.

Primary health care markets: the case of general dental services

Regulatory issues manifest themselves differently in other services. Here, we use the example of dentistry to illustrate these issues, particularly relating to umbrella regulation, on the basis that dentistry has developed into a mixed economy of both financing and provision. At least 20 per cent of general dentistry is now financed privately. In relation to consumer protection, four issues are noteworthy.

First, many adults and older people have to pay NHS user charges for dentistry, and therefore pay for both NHS and private services, so that payment is the norm. Payment for private dentistry has been little researched. A significant proportion is paid for through dental insurance or health cash plans (*see* Chapter 4). For Denplan, at least, dentists are expected to tell patients what the treatment will cost before it is carried out, and Denplan has told us that they monitor dentists to ensure that they do.

The main problem has less to do with private financing itself than with confusion between NHS and private payment. Because the same dentists generally offer both NHS and private treatment, and both attract charges, patients can be unclear whether they are being treated on the NHS or privately. (We understand that any one visit will almost always be either NHS or private, but there is no formal reason why a single visit should not involve both NHS and private treatment.) They may not be told how much treatment will cost before it is done – this is only now becoming formal government policy for the NHS, under the 2000 dental strategy.

In its dental strategy,[31] the Government has indicated that NHS dentists will be expected to tell patients what treatment they propose, and what it will cost. We hope that dentists will also be obliged to make it clear, up front, whether treatment is on the NHS or is private, and, if the former, what the NHS user charges will amount to. There could be regular mailings to people, or advertisements announcing scales of charges in newspapers. The move to basic consumer information under the dental strategy is welcome. A further step could be taken to require all dentists to inform patients about costs, whether NHS or private.

Second, general dentistry has until recently been neglected by the State. There appear to be differences between the quality of NHS and private dental work. NHS dentists have reported problems in delivering good-quality care for the money available within the NHS.[32] In addition, NHS dentistry has lagged behind general medical practice (itself relatively slow to develop such schemes) in the introduction of quality assurance and clinical governance. The introduction of clinical governance in dentistry was only announced in the dental strategy in 2000. A far as we can judge, dentists are often more closely monitored in private settings, by the insurers and the companies they work for, than in the NHS. Whether dentists work within the Denplan scheme, or work for Boots or one of the other chains, they are subjected to regular audit of the quality of their work. Taking the problems of NHS remuneration and the oversight of private work together, it seems likely that the quality of private dentistry is higher than in the NHS. We could not find any direct evidence to support this impression, but this view is shared by people we spoke to about it, as well as by patients, anecdotally. The central consumer issue concerns this difference in quality of treatment between the two sectors. The minimum action should be to seek to ensure that treatment in all settings is of a basic acceptable standard.

Third, as noted in Chapters 3 and 4, the growth of private financing and provision over the last few years has led to problems in access to NHS dentistry. The Government estimates that two million people who want one cannot find an NHS dentist.[33] It should be stressed that this is happening against a background of steadily improving oral health. For example, the average 12 year old had five decayed, missing or filled teeth in 1973, and just one or two in 1993.[34] Nevertheless, there is a real problem here, particularly for people on low income who qualify for exemptions from NHS user charges but who cannot find an NHS dentist to treat them, and who cannot afford full-cost private treatment. Put more bluntly, growing limitations in the funding of NHS general dental services have led to access problems, and even when patients go to an NHS dentist, the quality of care may be lower than in the private sector, in spite of the best efforts of those working within NHS dentistry.

Thus, access to services and quality are obvious foci for consumer-oriented regulation and changes to funding. It is notable that the Government's dental strategy contains only modest proposals to increase access, such as walk-in dental centres. The Government could increase the rates of payment for NHS work and thereby increase the supply of NHS dentistry. An integrated approach to regulation across NHS and private dentistry is a precursor to any solution to the access problem.

Fourth, a number of large firms, including Boots, own dental bodies corporate that offer salaried private dental services. They are an alternative organisational structure to the traditional general dental practice contracted to deliver services to the NHS. Having attracted relatively little commercial interest until recently, dentistry is now being used to create chains of outlets like those that have developed in optical services. Boots, for example, has announced an intention to create a large chain, possibly involving hundreds of outlets. The dental strategy recognises this interest, and the Government has hinted that it may permit the creation of more bodies corporate in the future, if there is demand for them.

However, that there are no proposals to regulate the services delivered by dental bodies corporate. If it is possible to increase the market for private dentistry, then private firms will do so. This may well reduce further the supply of dentists willing to do NHS work, and exacerbate problems of access and quality. A government committed to a good dental service for the whole population would need to regulate the activities of these bodies, so that they contributed to public as well as their own private goals. There is no sign at present that this is likely to happen.

Dentistry in the UK exhibits many of the problems and opportunities of public–private relations that may develop if the Government pursues its intention to encourage more private provision. The Government will need to maintain a clear focus on the problems that arise, and a willingness to regulate public and private services as part of a single system.

Conclusions

In this chapter, we have reviewed the regulation of the financing and provision of private health care. There have been some important positive developments in the last few years, but there is a lot still to be done. In relation to financing, the Competition Commission and OFT have both demonstrated that they are prepared to act in order to protect and promote consumer interests. The FSA is beginning its work, and it seems reasonable to hope that the 'partial umbrella' that it has created over private medical insurance and health cash plans will improve *ex ante* protections and the workings of complaints mechanisms.

However, an overall view of the regulation of the financing of private health care reveals a patchy picture. Private medical insurance remains subject to a mix of voluntary and statutory regulation. Improvements in its design and sales literature have depended on the work of the OFT, which cannot reasonably be expected to devote substantial resources to this sector indefinitely. The largest health cash provider (HSA) is not regulated by the FSA. The weakness of protections for people who pay cash for surgery suggests that an early review of financing is needed, as called for by the Health Committee.

Combining the observations made in this chapter with those made in Chapters 5 and 6, it is possible to identify policy changes that should be considered. Regulation could be developed to ensure that charges are transparent, particularly for people paying for their own treatment, so that consumers have the best understanding of likely costs. Ideally, insurers and providers would offer clearly defined packages for fixed prices – which we noted in Chapter 4 is already happening to some extent – and again further development in this direction should be encouraged by a regulator.

The current situation for provision of private health care is similar to that for financing. Recent developments suggest that the strength of regulation may be set to improve, as long as regulations under the Care Standards Act focus on services rather than premises. However, the Government's wider proposals for improving the quality of private health care remain vague. For example, there are no proposals yet that will directly address problems of the quality of clinical work in those areas where there is clear cause for concern, such as cosmetic surgery.

The Concordat, the Care Standards Act 2000, regulations and other policies need to be drawn together and given a focus. We think that one appropriate focus is consumer interests. The purpose of the Concordat should not be, as now, to make whatever local arrangements suit the NHS and private organisations. Instead, it should be to promote timely access to quality services, wherever they are provided. This might happen as a result of local action, but it would be far better if everyone understood that this was the driving force behind new policies. The dentistry case study was included precisely to address this point – local action to promote better access and coverage to general dental services is no substitute for central government action.

Finally, this chapter has re-emphasised the importance of breaking down boundaries between public and private sectors in order to assure good-quality services. The WHO World Health Report 2000[35] argues that the State has a responsibility to protect the interests of patients wherever they are treated. Thus, in the UK, the State should offer similar protections across all settings. To date, though, policy-making in England – and the UK more generally – has largely focused on the NHS.

The need now is to move towards more consistent regulation of services, so that regulations are similar, wherever the same services are provided and in whichever way they are financed. This means extending the concept of umbrella regulation used by the FSA. It will not be possible to have a single regulator for the whole of public and private health care in the near future, because professional regulation will continue to be separate, and because NHS and private regulation differ so markedly at the moment. However, there is a case for extending the FSA's role to include all aspects of private medical insurance and health cash plans. There could be also be umbrella regulation of the financing and provision of dentistry, since it is possible to treat it as a discrete service. There is no single fix here, as there will inevitably be areas where regulation of financial services intersects with the regulation of health care. All we can say, however, is that policy development needs to begin. There are some areas where the way forward is less obvious, notably for cash payment, as no appropriate regulator is available. But this only increases the need for a thorough review of regulation of private health care financing and provision.

In Chapters 5 and 6, it was stressed that other countries also regulate in order to ensure equitable financing or access to services, or both. In the next and last chapter, we analyse this other major objective for regulation – and the other major theme of this book.

References

1 Rice T. *The Economics of Health Reconsidered*. Chicago: Health Administration Press, 1998.
2 House of Commons Health Committee. *Regulation of Private and Other Independent Health Care*. Vol I. London: Stationery Office, 1999.

3   Rice T. *The Economics of Health Reconsidered*. Chicago: Health Administration Press, 1998.

4   Department of Social Security. *A New Contract for Welfare: partnership in pensions*. London: DSS, 1998.

5   Financial Services Authority. *Pensions Review Phase 2: report on the production and outcome of the advertising campaign*. London: FSA, 1999.

6   *Competition Act 1998*. London: Stationery Office, 1998.

7   *Private Health Insurance*. London: OFT, 1996.

8   *Private Health Insurance. Second Report*. London: OFT, 1998: 4

9   Ibid.: 6

10 Office of Fair Trading. *Private medical insurance and PMS markets are competitive says OFT but better information for policyholders is needed*. (Press release.) London: OFT, 1999.

11 Office of Fair Trading. *Health insurers improve consumer information*. London: OFT, 2000: 2

12 Ibid.: 3

13 The Insurance Ombudsman Bureau. *Annual Report 1998*. London: IOB, 1999.

14 Baldwin R. *Rules and Government*. Oxford: Clarendon Press, 1995: 1–15

15 Laing and Buisson. *Laing's Healthcare Market Review 1999–2000*. London: Laing and Buisson, 1999.

16 Department of Health. *The NHS Plan: a plan for investment; a plan for reform*. Cm 4818-I. London: Stationery Office, 2000.

17 Health Committee. *The Regulation of Private and Other Independent Healthcare*. Session 1998–99. 281-I. London: Stationery Office, 1999.

18 Association of Friendly Socities. *The Historical Context of Friendly Societies*. London: Association of Friendly Societies. October 1998.

19 BUPA. *Shaping the Future NHS. Long Term Planning for Hospitals and Related Services*. London: BUPA, 2000.

20 Secretary of State for Health. *The NHS Plan*. Cm 4818-I. London: Department of Health, 2000.

21 Health Committee. *The Regulation of Private and Other Independent Healthcare*. HC 281-I, Session 1998–99. London: Stationery Office, 1999.

22 Department of Health. *Regulation of Private and Independent Health Care*. London: DoH, 1999.

23 Milburn A. *Reinventing Health Care. A Modern NHS versus a Private Alternative*. Speech at the London School of Economics. London, 20 December 1999.

24 Keen J. *Private Health Care – No Longer a Pariah*. Interview with Gisela Stuart MP. Parliamentary Brief, January 2000: 16–18.

25 Department of Health. *Independent Health Care: national minimum standards regulations*. London: Department of Health, 2001.

26 *Discipline of Hospital Practitioners Bill*. London: Stationery Office, 2000.

27 General Medical Council. *Maintaining Good Medical Practice*. London: GMC, 1998.

28 Klein R. Regulating the medical profession: doctors and the public interest. In: Harrison A, editor. *Health Care UK 1997/98*. London: King's Fund, 1998: 13–25.

29 Chief Medical Officer. *Supporting Doctors, Protecting Patients*. London: Department of Health, 1998.

30 Salter B. *Medical Regulation and Public Trust*. London: King's Fund, 2000: 41.

31 Department of Health. *Modernising NHS Dentistry – Implementing the NHS Plan*. London: Department of Health, 2000.

32 Taylor-Gooby P, Sylvester S, Calnan M, Manley G. Knights, knaves and gnashers: professional values and private dentistry. *J Soc Policy* 2000; 29: 375–95.

33 Department of Health. *The NHS Plan – Modernising NHS Dentistry*. London: Department of Health, 2000.

34 WHO. *World Health Report 2000*. Geneva: WHO, 2000.

35 Ibid.

Chapter 8

Improving equity

Public–private relationships: the argument thus far

This book has focused mainly on public–private boundaries in health service delivery and financing, in order to identify some of the anomalies and inequities these relationships create. As a result, it is possible to lose sight of the fact that financing and access to health care in the UK are relatively equitable when judged against many other countries. As an illustration, the UK was ranked in the group of countries between 8th and 11th in the world out of 191 countries on 'fairness of financial contribution' in the WHO *World Health Report 2000*,[1] principally because the NHS is largely financed out of general tax revenue. On disability-adjusted life expectancy, the UK was ranked 14th in the world in terms of the level of its 'burden of disease', but second in terms of the distribution of that 'burden'. In other words, perhaps surprisingly, the population of the UK had one of the most equal distributions of life expectancy adjusted for disability in the world. The UK health system was ranked 18th overall when other measures of performance such as system 'responsiveness' were also taken into account.

Thus, the reasonably good, if still not excellent, rating for equity of financial contribution disguises issues that need tackling. For example, relatively long waits for elective surgery in the public sector, among other things, meant that the UK was ranked only in the mid-20s in terms of system 'responsiveness' (a subjective measure of the degree to which the system meets public expectations in terms of aspects like prompt attention, amenities, choice, dignity, confidentiality and autonomy). The WHO report emphasises the responsibility of the State for the fairness of financing, equity of access and quality of health care in both the private and public sectors. The main argument of this book is that current public–private relationships for 'final' (i.e. received by patients) health care goods and services in the UK need to be critically reviewed. Most of the relationships have developed in an *ad hoc* fashion over many years, and their consequences have not been subjected to serious examination. This final chapter summarises the issues raised in the course of the last seven chapters in relation to equity of financing and access to health services, using them to identify priorities for policy-making, and setting our arguments in a broader context of policy-making for public–private relations.

In Chapter 1 we noted that relatively little policy attention was paid to the private health care sector and its relationship with the NHS before 1999. This had been the case in spite of evidence that consumer interests were not always adequately promoted or protected, and problems of coverage and access created by the presence of a private system running alongside the NHS. The situation is changing. Since 1999, the Labour Government has indicated its intention to act in order to protect patients' interests and to improve equity of financing, coverage and access. Some of these intentions may not be translated into firm actions, but some will, so now is a good time to review where we are and make policy proposals for the future. In addition, the Government has promised the largest ever increase in public funding for health care, which should allow unprecedented scope for improving the equity of financing and coverage of health services in the UK.

The book has outlined the contours of public–private relations, and the unregulated growth of many types of private health care alongside the NHS. The private health care sector is substantial, accounting for at least 16 per cent of UK health care expenditure. Private medical insurance and private acute hospital care have attracted most comment from the media and policy analysts, but the private sector is more extensive and more varied than these commentaries suggest. For example, there is a substantial private pharmaceutical market, and a wide range of private primary care services, including dentistry and optical services.

There are different balances between public and private financing and provision depending on the sector or service in question. Private medical insurance and self-payment account for some 16 per cent of total expenditure on acute hospital care. The proportions are higher for specific services. For example, around 20 per cent of general dentistry, over 40 per cent of eyesight tests and around 95 per cent of complementary therapies are financed privately. Sometimes the location of a public–private boundary is the result of conscious government action, as in the case of optical services under both Conservative and Labour governments. More often, though, boundaries have developed disjointedly and incrementally over time, with their locations determined by a number of factors, including the willingness and ability of people to pay for services, the desire of professionals to maintain private practices and the perceptions of successive governments concerning the legitimate scope of state financing or regulation.

The consequences of having a private sector alongside the NHS have moved up the policy agenda in the last very few years, and particularly since the 2001 General Election. These consequences are manifested as problems of financing, coverage and access to services – and we focus on them here.

The challenge facing government

Rawls' difference principle, described in Chapter 1, suggests that it is acceptable for individuals to have different basic talents or resources, and to use them in different ways, as long as they do not unduly disadvantage other members of a society. In the case of health care, Daniels and colleagues[2] argue that one person's use of a good or service should not unduly inconvenience or harm anyone else's ability to use it. As we have seen, some current health service arrangements violate this equity principle, principally where payment buys preferential access to services, and particularly where these services are provided by the same people who also provide publicly financed services.

In considering the consequences, the central dilemma facing all governments in the UK is how to balance individual choice with the goal of greater equity in health care within available public resources. Governments are faced with powerful professions that are committed to retaining their right to practise both publicly and privately, and better-off people who want to be able to buy private treatment, believing it to be of better quality. It is almost certainly not possible to outlaw private practice entirely, if only because the degree of coercion required on the part of government. Equally, providing tax breaks to encourage higher take-up of private medical insurance is inequitable and also likely to be inefficient – and the Labour Government has ruled it out in the NHS Plan, effectively taking it off the political agenda. The Government has, therefore, to engage in a more subtle balancing act, determining whether there is scope for a slightly different balance of priorities, and the risks and benefits of such a move.

The task, then, is to consider ways in which equity can be increased within these constraints. In the next section the equity effects of new Labour Government policies are assessed. These are followed by our proposals for policies that future governments could consider on financing, coverage and access.

Trends in Labour Government policy

Private finance for services

The NHS Plan devoted a chapter to alternative methods of financing health care, in the course of which it presented strong arguments against extending the use of private medical insurance in the UK. The document noted the inequities that can result from its use for both the financing and provision of services. (Presumably the arguments extend to other forms of private health insurance such as for dental care – though the NHS Plan does not state that this is the case.) This stance is supported by wider changes in government policy, including increases in taxation of private medical insurance.

In similar vein, the Labour-aligned Institute for Public Policy Research (IPPR) report produced by its Commission on Public Private Partnerships restated the case for universal health services financed from general taxation, basing its argument on the criteria of social justice (equity), efficiency and democracy.[3] While the IPPR Commission advocated an open-minded approach to deciding whether public *provision* was superior to the private or voluntary sectors in different sectors and for different purposes, it did not equivocate over public *finance* in key areas such as education and health. As the Commission put it:

> The reason we are interested in PPPs [public private partnerships] is because we want to explore all possible avenues for increasing the quality and responsiveness of publicly funded services. Services that are universal and free at the point of use form a central part of our commitment to social justice, economic efficiency and democratic accountability.[4]

Thus, the Government will not actively encourage the use of private medical insurance or other sources of private financing for access to services at any point in the foreseeable future. Yet the Government has not pursued policies directly to restrict the uptake of private insurance save for taxing it like other forms of insurance. Similarly, it has not designed any new policies specifically to address financing issues arising from self-payment or other forms of payment such as health cash plans. Instead, it has pursued a series of inter-linked policies aimed at strengthening the public system, one consequence of which could be a reduction in the need for privately financed health care.

Strengthening the public system

The Government's proposals in this respect indicate a clear direction of travel and key policies are outlined in the following paragraphs.

On the issue of the NHS *workforce*, which has also moved up the policy agenda over the last few years, there are ambitious plans to increase the number of hospital medical specialists, GPs, nurses, theatre sessions and beds in order to raise the capacity of the Service significantly. The extra resources and staff are linked to standards and targets, designed particularly to increase the responsiveness of the Service to its patients (perhaps the WHO rankings provided a stimulus in this respect). For example, the NHS Plan sets out a target reduction in maximum waits for outpatient appointments of three months and inpatient admissions of six months, with two-thirds of appointments to be pre-booked by 2003/04.

The Government has taken steps to expand some aspects of *coverage* in order to remove inequities and to restrict others in a number of services. Part 4 of the NHS Act 2000 restored free nursing care to nursing home patients, on the basis of a joint health and social care assessment of their needs. Free NHS nursing care will be extended to people living at home, again subject to an assessment. The Government has not gone as far as it could have done in this respect, and made all personal care free, but it has nevertheless taken a step towards restoring nursing coverage for older people. Free eyesight tests were restored for people aged 60 years and over, leading to a marked increase in the proportion of all tests undertaken that were free to users. The tax deductibility of private medical insurance premiums for people over 60 years has been removed. There are also plans for the NHS to extend its involvement in occupational health services that are largely private at present.

It may seem strange that general dentistry was not among the services to which coverage was extended in order to make it more equitable. The NHS dental strategy was published in the wake of the NHS Plan in the Autumn of 2000. It recognised that general dentistry is not available in all parts of the UK, and that this results in problems of access in some areas. The strategy did not address coverage issues created by the presence of a significant private sector and focused mainly on policies for existing NHS services. It is unclear why dentistry is deemed to be different to eyesight tests. It could be that the Government – in spite of Mr Blair's statements to the contrary – simply does not want to spend more public money on this part of the NHS (and dentistry costs the State more than eye tests).

Similarly, the Government has not chosen to review or alter the pattern of co-payments and exemptions that apply to GP pharmaceuticals. This may be because of the extent of exemptions (e.g. for people receiving welfare benefits) and the cost of reductions in user charges. Indeed, it is apparent that the Government continues to have worries about the overall cost of the Service and has developed new institutional responses to the perennial problem of appropriate cost containment (perhaps precisely *because* it has determined significantly to extend the coverage of the NHS – for example, into costly long-term care). For example, the National Institute for Clinical Excellence (NICE) has the responsibility of advising the NHS and its purchasers on which new treatments and pharmaceuticals are likely to be the most effective and cost-effective to provide publicly. Yet, its decision to limit the use of Cox 2 Inhibitors to serious cases appears to have been influenced primarily by considerations of their cost rather than their cost-effectiveness.[5] As the scope of the NHS expands (e.g. in long-term care and eye screening), there is no reason why restrictions of coverage should not increase in other areas (e.g. in the case of new drugs).

The Labour Government has also introduced new policies and legislation on *quality*. The series of responses to the Bristol Royal Infirmary case, including the commitment to develop clinical governance to assure the quality of care offered by NHS providers and the moves to assure the public that professionals' competence is maintained and checked periodically, are all designed to raise public confidence in and support for a publicly financed, universal health system. It will be difficult to attain the ambitious vision for the future of the NHS painted in the Bristol inquiry: 'The culture of the future must be a culture of safety and quality; a culture of openness and accountability; a culture of public service; a culture in which collaborative teamwork is prized; and a culture of flexibility in which innovation can flourish in response to patients' needs.'[6] However, there is little doubt that 'Bristol', as it is now known, has entirely altered the Service's and the Government's attitude to resourcing, setting standards, improving management, monitoring the quality of services and holding professionals accountable for the quality of what they do. While these new policies are not directly concerned with equity of access, they would, if successful, improve the standard of services in the public sector, thereby reducing the need for people to use private provision.

The Government has taken some important steps to reduce the negative effects on the NHS and its patients of the existence of a parallel private surgical sector in which many NHS surgeons have a personal financial interest. Thus, the Government proposes to change the current pattern of medical specialist contracts with the NHS so that full-time consultants will be rewarded commensurately for their entire commitment to the public system.

There are also proposals to tie some part of specialists' remuneration to their level of productivity in the NHS, perhaps with floors and/or targets for performance in line with the wider goals of the Service.

The Government has also signed a Concordat with the private health care sector, which formalises the ability of the NHS to make greater use of private sector facilities. This appears to be motivated primarily by a desire to increase the volume of elective surgery carried out on behalf of the NHS by making use of private centres specialising in bulk production of relatively routine procedures such as hip replacements and hernia repairs, thereby improving public patients' access to precisely those services that motivate the better-off to purchase care privately.

We may well see greater NHS use of private hospitals or specialist clinics in future, possibly through government-sanctioned selective contracting-out of services that private hospitals are able to provide safely and cost-effectively, such as cataract operations and other day surgical procedures. As long as the shift of provision out of NHS hospitals does not adversely affect the ability of public hospitals to provide their remaining essential services (for which there is no private equivalent), then the Concordat is likely to be neutral or better in terms equity of access than previous arrangements. The only change will be the location of treatment.

We note, though, that the Concordat stresses that co-ordination will be carried out locally rather than nationally. Therefore, the Government is eschewing a regulatory role, and will not seek to achieve any particular balance of public and private provision. The precise effects of such contracting-out to the private sector will depend on the nature of the contracts between the NHS and the private providers, particularly the ability of the NHS to control who gets treated and on what terms, so that the private sector is unable to provide just one part of a treatment or select easier and less costly cases, leaving the remainder for the NHS.

Overall, then, the Labour Government has begun to create a new policy framework for parts of the private health sector and key public–private relationships.

Reducing remaining inequities

The Labour Government's concerted change of policy direction makes it possible to have a serious debate about the sources of inequity produced by public–private relationships. As recently as 1998, a proposal to review public–private relations might have seemed naive, but the Government has now placed private health care firmly on the policy agenda and appears willing to increase the level of public funding of the NHS in order fundamentally to alter the inevitable trade-offs between individual choice, equity and the total cost of publicly financed services.

The overseas' experiences discussed in Chapters 5 and 6 were chosen to exemplify the complexities of public policy responses to public–private mixtures of finance, particularly when the goal is equity. The Dutch have largely succeeded in reconciling mixed finance with equity, but only through constant vigilance and repeated policy responses to inequities as they arise. For example, when more affluent, older citizens in the private sector were being charged much more than they could handle, measures were instituted requiring the rest of the population of private insurees to help them out financially. Another example is the regulation to prevent privately insured patients from gaining undue advantage in the queue for elective surgery, which is unheard of in the UK. All in all, these experiences show that it is possible, but not easy, to devise policies and regulations for private health care – or for the public and private sectors as a whole – in pursuit of equity goals. Indeed, such regulations can lead to arrangements that are more equitable overall than those in the UK, with its parallel public and private sectors.

The lack of comparable regulation in the UK over the use of private medical insurance and self-payment makes access to key services less equitable, as measured in terms of public and private patients' surgical waiting times. Similar arguments apply in the case of dentistry. Yet the evidence from overseas shows that different trade-offs are possible. The Netherlands, for example, has a fairer system in terms of access, but probably more inequitable financing. In general, then, society and government needs to decide which equity goal or goals to pursue, how vigorously and for which services. To us, public financing and universality of key services is fundamental if services are to be equitable, as well as efficient. Issues of public versus private or voluntary sector provision are strictly secondary, albeit important in specific instances. Hence, proposals affecting financing are discussed first, before coverage and access.

Proposals for more equitable financing

The experience of both the UK and the other countries studied in this book shows that it is extremely difficult, if not impossible, for private financing to co-exist fairly with a public system unless the advantages of 'double-cover' insurance and direct payment are largely eliminated. In a parallel public and private system, it is inevitable that private insurers and providers will make available selective provision while leaving the sickest people and most unprofitable services for the public sector to provide,[7] unless, like the Dutch, private insurance is strictly regulated to be community-rated and thereby relatively more equitable.

Confining private financing to supplementary services

Following the above analysis, one potential policy response to the current inequity of financing, and thereby of access, generated by the UK parallel public–private arrangements, would be to forbid private payment and insurance for all health services covered by the NHS. The example of Canada could be followed, which confines private financing of services to a purely supplementary private health care option. Thus, the boundary between a public sector focused on equity of finance and access and a private sector that reflects individuals' preferences for the use of their discretionary income, would become far clearer. In these circumstances, it should be possible to determine precisely which sorts of health care advantages people with higher incomes should be permitted to secure. The advantages could be confined to highly discretionary treatments and hotel services, or they could be broader. In any event, they would have to be services not covered by the public scheme.

In some ways, there is a *de facto* trend in this direction. The current government is expanding capacity for universal coverage within the NHS. At the same time, private medical insurance is facing problems of adverse selection, resulting in more risk-rating and more conditional coverage. As a result, the private sector may well see its future in providing top-up and supplementary services (perhaps increasingly paid for out-of-pocket), plus more elective provision for public patients on contract to the NHS.

A comprehensive private 'opt-out'

A quite different means of eliminating 'double cover' that would increase the market for private medical insurance would be to permit people who could afford it to remove themselves (with some level of tax rebate) from coverage by the NHS in return for taking out comprehensive private health care insurance so that they would not need to use the public system at all. The tax rebate would have to be set in such a way that those exiting continued to make an adequate contribution towards the costs of the services of those who remained under the NHS. A wider-ranging, compulsory variant of this approach would see publicly financed health care reserved for people below a specified income, with extensive regulation to ensure that the publicly financed system was fairly funded for the needs of the people it served. Such models based on public finance for the less well-off and private arrangements for better-off people would be substantially less equitable than the Canadian-style approach discussed above, but the resultant inequities would be clearly apparent.

Such a system could be organised to retain redistributive financing, either by setting the tax rebate at such a level that better-off people were still substantially contributing to the health care of less well-off people, or by requiring additional contributions as part of private insurance to be used to subsidise the publicly financed sector, as in the Netherlands. Indeed, if the scale of any tax reductions offered to better-off people that accompanied the change from current arrangements was carefully calculated (i.e. was not too great), the shift to an explicitly 'two-tier' system could lead to an increase in the level and quality of care in the new public sector relative to the newly expanded private sector.

Much of the impact on equity would depend on the standard of services and access levels in the publicly financed system and the amount of tax paid by the better-off towards the health services of those covered publicly, since those least able to pay for themselves are most likely to require services. There is always the risk that the *per capita* public funds available to those reliant on the public sector could fall under such an arrangement and be raised disproportionately from those on lower incomes if the tax concessions to the better-off are too generous. Furthermore, at least initially, there would be substantial 'dead weight costs', as the foregone government income from tax relief would go disproportionately to people who already have private insurance or who could easily afford it but who currently choose to pay out-of-pocket.

With these concerns in mind, David Green's proposal for 'stakeholder health insurance' is based on the idea of a government guarantee of a standard of coverage in the NHS equivalent to the personal market choices of middle-income earners, thereby ensuring that those unable to afford private insurance would not be consigned to a residual or second-class service.[8] One difficulty with this would be sustaining such a guarantee over time in a two-tier system, as governments change and economic circumstances shift. This approach would also tie what was provided from public sources to the coverage and service choices of middle-income people and their insurers, with no assurance that these represented the best value-for-money from the perspective of a public scheme. To work well, this proposal would depend on the total public and private spending on health services in the UK rising (as would the previous approach). Furthermore, it is not at all self-evident that spending more on health services would be the best means of improving health or reducing health inequalities compared with measures outside the health sector, such as improvements in education in deprived neighbourhoods and benefit changes to reduce child poverty.[9,10]

Implementation issues in removing 'double cover'

Despite their potential drawbacks, both the 'Canadian' and the 'opt-out', or 'two-tier', option are worth including in any future discussion of the financing of health care in the UK. Although they represent a major change from current arrangements (for example, they would have huge implications for provider organisations), they do offer the potential to make the co-existence of private insurance and public financing work more fairly and more clearly than the current blurred and inconsistent arrangements, in which the ostensible goals of equity of financing, access and use are regularly flouted by the existence of a relatively unregulated, parallel, privately financed health care sector.

However, there is no doubt that there would be many practical difficulties to overcome in implementing either the 'two-tier' or the strictly supplementary private sector model in the UK. The 'Canadian' approach would require a clear NHS/non-NHS boundary to be drawn, most likely accompanied by an increase in the level of funding of the public system so that reasonable access terms could be assured in the compulsory universal system. Of course, even with higher levels of public finance, it is likely that there would be constant pressure in a Canadian-style system from better-off individuals and private interests to bend the rules preventing 'double-cover' private provision, and to blur the clarity and simplicity of the new system. One way to reduce this pressure would be to continue to increase spending in the public system. Yet, it is entirely possible that governments would have other priorities for scarce tax resources and that health spending could 'crowd out' other more beneficial social spending.

In the case of the other option of a public system for only part of the population, the first major task would be to determine the income cut-off, which would distinguish publicly from privately financed patients if there were a compulsory separation between the two, rather than one based on individual choice. Over the longer term, any government would need to guard against the risk of reductions in the real level of funding of the public system for those on lower incomes, since higher earners could well become increasingly reluctant to pay for a health care system they did not use. It would be imperative to devise a system of funding for the public system that accounted fairly for the higher level of health care needed *per capita* likely in the publicly served population. This is not a trivial problem.

Regulation to make private insurance more equitable

Regardless of these options, there is a need to change the regulations governing private medical insurance in order to make it more equitable than it is today. Such reforms should be seriously considered even if none of the major changes to the relations between the NHS and the private sector discussed above occur. Indeed, the history of Western health care systems shows that major, system-wide change is the exception rather than the rule, irrespective of the strength of the case, since it requires an exceptional conjunction of favourable circumstances both outside and within the health sector.[11] Both the 'Canadian' model and the 'two-tier' model discussed above would amount to a revolution in the UK health care system comparable with the inception of the NHS. Seen in this light, it is unlikely that a sufficiently strong coalition of support, linked to supportive external conditions, will come about to allow either model to be introduced, irrespective of their merits. Thus, other, more realistic responses to managing the choice–equity dilemma will need to be developed.

One such proposal, designed to allow private payment to continue in its current form but to limit its negative effects, would be to require that coverage in private health insurance policies should include all reasonable aspects of diagnosing and treating a problem. As was noted in Chapters 3 and 4, some guaranteed packages are already offered by insurers. These should include follow-up care and coverage for any adverse effects or complications during the following period (e.g. a month). This whole-package approach protects consumers as well as the NHS from footing the bills for parts of private care or for things that go wrong. It can also prevent better-off patients slipping informally between public and private sectors during the course of a treatment in order to derive overall advantage from both sectors. It should also be required when private practitioners price their work for patients paying in cash rather than using insurance.

In order to improve equity specifically within the private insurance market, the Government could require age-of-entry community-rating in private medical insurance, eliminating the risk-rating of premiums. We believe that the experiences in Ireland analysed in Chapter 6 are helpful here. The Irish Advisory Group has recommended age-of-entry community-rating, in which each person's lifetime premium is set by the age at which they begin to subscribe. If someone drops out and re-enters later, they pay the higher rate according to the age at which they re-enter. This scheme provides incentives for young adults to sign on early and keep their coverage, so their lifetime rate will be low and not rise in real terms, except as necessary to reflect the general rise in medical costs. Setting community rates by age of entry was also the principal conclusion of the Australian Commission that deliberated about fair markets in health insurance.[12] A similar approach is worthy of discussion in the UK, as a means of preventing adverse selection in insurance and premium hikes for older people.

We further recommend guaranteed enrolment for older people and setting a maximum waiting time, during which treatment of pre-existing conditions can legitimately be excluded from coverage. We also recommend that prices for private medical insurance policies and private charges for procedures and services are required to be posted on a consistent, comparable basis so that people can make sensible choices between insurers and private providers. In similar vein, we recommend that public information be made available on the performance of private insurers (e.g. percentage of claims settled within a particular time) and quality of care delivered by different private hospitals.

Supplementary mutual funds

Both the 'Canadian' and 'opt-out' models discussed above would appear to work better (i.e. more equitably) with increases in spending on health services. One proposal to increase the level of overall funding, if employers or communities so wished, would be to supplement public finance from local sources. Usually, increases in non-governmental sources of finance for health care increase inequity since they rarely benefit the entire population (e.g. out-of-pocket payment and private insurance). By contrast, supplementary mutual funds (SMFs) are one potential form of non-governmental support for the NHS and other health services providers, which may increase overall funding while minimising adverse consequences for equity. Indeed, supplementary funding from mutual sources might even replace privately financed treatment with a more equitable and affordable arrangement.

Although the current government and the Treasury seem confident that comprehensive health care can continue to be universally provided from general taxation (albeit with some user charges), a number of observers worry that current public funding may become increasingly inadequate to support the NHS to a sufficient standard to maintain a reasonable degree of equity between those who can and cannot purchase additional private care.[13] Higher standards of clinical excellence throughout the NHS, rapid advances in medical and genetic science, increased costs of implementing the NHS Plan (e.g. from large increases in the clinical workforce), the capital costs of repairing or replacing old hospitals and building new health centres, and the increased costs of recruiting and retaining clinical staff, may drive costs up faster than gains in effectiveness and productivity. One need not choose sides in this debate, however, to consider future options for new forms of non-governmental funding. As we have documented, patients' savings or their private insurance already fund health care services substantially in some areas, such as long-term care and waiting list surgery. Thus, the comprehensiveness of public funding is already something of a myth, though the NHS is still remarkable in the range of services it does provide for one of the lowest *per capita* public budgets in Europe.

Supplementary mutual funds (SMFs) are different to 'private' funds in the usual sense of the term, since they are collective, non-governmental schemes. SMFs cover a class of contributory schemes that, while not insurance, are non-profit subscriptions for quick access to a specified range of specialist health services. In this respect they have some characteristics in common with health cash plans discussed in Chapters 1 and 4. One traditional form in the period before the NHS was the 'Hospital Saturday Fund' that supported local hospitals through small weekly contributions that most workers could afford. In return, they could get access to a wide array of hospital services. Besides being non-profit, SMFs could support and strengthen the local NHS hospital or other service rather than supporting private hospitals that can weaken the NHS. It is instructive to read how Sir Ronald Matthews contrasted such contributory schemes with insurance policies in 1935.[14] A contributory scheme, he wrote, 'should make direct appeal to every class in the community and should provide for the widest possible representation within itself so that by co-operation and pooling of resources (those for whom no treatment is required paying to some extent for the others), we create a standard, symbolic contributor who may be able to pay for himself and … his dependants'. Sir Ronald envisioned a nation of democratically governed, user-based associations, fundamentally different from insurance. With insurance a person looks out only for himself/herself, while in a voluntary association people help each other. 'Reciprocity seems to be the most complete answer and foil to insurance,' he noted.

The idea of SMFs in one form or another contains echoes of New Labour's rhetoric of public–private partnerships, mutual co-operation and self-help. Employers or unions could sponsor SMFs, and they could be tied to an occupational health programme designed to minimise time off work due to sickness. Employers would find such a fund much cheaper and more equitable than private insurance, and it could apply to all employees. Participation at these low rates could be voluntary or mandatory. A SMF could also be sponsored by a broader organisation, such as a business association or a town council. Health authorities or primary care trusts could also sponsor SMFs if their 'publicfunding only' outlook and regulatory restrictions did not prohibit them. It would be important as far as possible to guard against the existence of SMFs managed by NHS bodies being used by governments as a reason for reducing the rate of increase of mainstream NHS funding (there may be lessons to be learned from the recent experience of the NHS and National Lottery funding in this regard). By contrast, the current public policies and regulations over non-governmental financing principally benefit the insurance companies, because they block more user-based, participatory alternatives, while allowing insurers to 'cherry pick' whom they wish to insure, and what they wish to cover them for.

The attractiveness of SMFs depends on the value placed on additional health services spending and the desire for services beyond those paid for from general taxation. SMFs inevitably have drawbacks. For example, the advent of SMFs in different parts of the country could lead to divergence between areas in the availability of health care funding. Whether this was regarded as desirable would depend on governmental and wider public priorities. In addition, flat-rate contributions, however modest, would represent a more regressive form of financing than general taxation used currently to support most NHS spending. On the other hand, SMFs could conceivably be structured around progressive contributions, although this would not be easy. A key feature is that contributions should be community-rated and not discriminate by age or health condition. SMFs depend on broad participation centred on the working population (like tax-financed systems).

Despite these potential limitations, we can see merits in further exploration of the role of SMFs in the UK as a less-inequitable alternative to current forms of private financing of services. Applying the 'benchmarks of fairness'[15] described in Chapter 1 to SMFs, a comparison with other forms of private finance for services suggests that they score well without being as fair as taxes (*see* Table 8.1).

Table 8.1 Scores on 'benchmarks of inequity'* of different forms of non-governmental financing for health services

Source of finance	B1	B2	B3	B4	B5	Total inequity score
Current out-of-pocket private care	5	5	5	5	5	25
Fair market out-of-pocket private care	5	4	5	5	4	23
Current private health insurance	4	3	4	3	3	17
Fair market private health insurance	3	2	3	3	2	13
Supplementary mutual funds	2	1	2	2	1	8

* Benchmarks scored from 0 (least inequitable) to 5 (most inequitable), maximum inequity score = 25

B1 = To what extent does the policy make universal access and participation more inequitable or less so?

B2 = To what extent does the policy make coverage for services more inequitable or less so?

B3 = To what degree are contributions and coverage based on health risk?

B4 = To what extent do payments depend on ability to pay?

B5 = To what extent does the policy increase or minimise non-financial barriers to access to services?

Making coverage more equitable: user charges

There are anomalies in what is free and what is charged for under the NHS, which affect equitable coverage and financing. We have set out the mosaic of out-of-pocket and NHS user charges (co-payments) for a range of services in previous chapters. International evidence suggests that user charges can deter people on lower incomes from accessing services when they need them, as well as deterring use of appropriate and inappropriate care equally.[16] Charges also cost to collect, account for and adjudicate, regardless of their size. They can distract clinical staff from the delivery of care and interfere in relations between clinicians and patients. For these reasons, some countries make very limited use of them.

While none of the current anomalies may present major difficulties for a patient, inconsistencies and illogicalities in what is and is not covered are worthy of attention. For example, why should someone who has suffered the indignity of hair loss through chemotherapy or other treatment be expected to pay £29.50 for a wig, as the NHS currently requires? Does anyone really believe that the charge deters frivolous consumption or that the wig is not an integral part of the treatment? If no good reason can be found for this charge then it should be removed and wigs made free. Alternatively, if the wig is regarded as purely cosmetic and not an essential part of the medical care of the individual, patients should be expected to buy it entirely out-of-pocket.

The example of the current government restoring free eyesight tests for people aged 60 years and over shows that the Labour Government has the will and the resources to reverse the previous narrowing of the scope of the NHS in certain service areas, by removing user charges. However, the fact remains that other entitlements to NHS services – whether free or charged for – are still not clear or consistent. For example, entitlement to free GP pharmaceuticals without a co-payment is assessed on the basis of a complicated mix of age, reliance on welfare benefits and clinical status. There is little intellectual coherence underlying this regime.

These observations lead to two broad policy options. The first option is to acknowledge that some services will continue as a mix of NHS, means-tested and private provision, but develop a more consistent basis for deciding who has to pay for services, and what they should pay for, as is beginning to occur in the long-term care of older people. This option appears to work already for well-defined services such as general optical services, but it is less attractive where the mix of services is more complicated, as it is in dentistry and long-term care.

The second option is to introduce, or restore, free services to everyone who 'needs' them – which would also provide the consistency that is currently missing. That is, the universal principle would be applied in order to guarantee equitable coverage. This is effectively what the Government has done by restoring free eyesight tests for people aged 60 years and over. We cannot think of any compelling argument for stopping there, aside from the cost. One way of making progress, taking resource constraints into account, would be to remove user charges for the most cost-effective GP pharmaceuticals and other services first. In addition, the level of remaining NHS user charges should be kept under regular review.

In general dentistry, removal of user charges would be necessary but not sufficient, because dentists are reluctant to treat patients at current levels of payment. The Government will either have to increase the levels of payment for NHS work, or change the current dental contract to require all dentists to provide a basic NHS service. To date, the Government has taken neither course.

Making access more equitable

In practice, some financing issues manifest themselves to patients as access problems, and these are most apparent in the case of non-urgent hospital services. For elective hospital treatment, private sector access is based on ability to pay rather than clinical need paid for from public funds. Arguments about NHS funding levels and their relation to waiting times are important, but tend to obscure the simpler point that private health care allows access to private elective care on the basis of ability to pay rather than clinical need. On the other hand, the more the NHS works to reduce waits in the public sector, the smaller the advantage of private access to elective surgery. We recommend a number of policy changes to improve equity of access.

Eliminate perverse incentives

Access to elective services in the public sector is shaped as much by the precise structure of the relationships between the parallel public and private sectors as by the level of funding for electives. Current arrangements generate perverse incentives for surgeons in the NHS with private practices to minimise the number of public patients they treat, maximise NHS waiting times, and encourage the view among patients that the only way to receive timely treatment is to pay for it privately.[17] The existence of these perverse incentives says nothing about the motivation of individual surgeons, many of whom work hard for the NHS, but demonstrates how poorly current arrangements generally support a high level of productivity in the public sector.

In order to minimise the perverse incentives in the current system, the following require modification:

- the NHS maximum part-time specialist salaried contract without productivity targets that encourages publicly trained and paid specialists to build up a private practice on the access to patients, professional networks and resources of the public system
- the practice of permitting the same specialists to manage their own waiting lists
- permitting long-term shortages to evolve in many specialties and strict control of public sector operating capacity

- allowing many NHS surgeons to spend as little as four to six hours a week operating on NHS patients.[18,19,20,21]

As noted above, the Government has made a range of policy proposals to tackle these issues.

There is also a need to manage the sequence of events from first referral to treatment far more actively. Currently, surgeons and other specialists manage thousands of little pools in each specialty and hospital, into which they toss or fish out patients treading water while they wait, according to highly variable and unaccountable criteria. This *ad hoc* arrangement, which invites variable treatment thresholds and manipulation, needs to be replaced by co-ordinated management of the patient's entire clinical journey through the system, from initial referral to final treatment, if appropriate. Fortunately, first steps are being taken in this direction through a number of pilot priority scoring and booking schemes in various parts of the country. Area-wide referral and booking systems are being developed, along with the criteria required to manage each stage in the patient's progress. After a long period of development, a national surgical booking system now operates in New Zealand, covering many of the commonest waiting list procedures such as coronary artery bypass grafts, hip and knee replacements, and cataract removals.[22] Given the close similarities between the UK and New Zealand in the relations between the public and private sectors for elective surgery, much can and is being learned from this model for the NHS.

Minimise distortions created by private practice

Closer control and separation of NHS doctors' private practices from their public work are also needed. Hospital consultants, for example, should only be allowed to undertake private work once they have met agreed targets for numbers of NHS patients treated, or other performance measures to ensure that their private work does not affect their NHS work. Such policy changes are already under consideration and would also protect specialists from accusations of conflicts of interest. Nonetheless, it is hard to use waiting time targets for regulatory purposes since they are open to extensive manipulation and are also affected by circumstances outside the surgeon's control, such as GP referral habits. The Government's proposal to impose a seven-year moratorium on new NHS consultants' freedom to undertake private practice recognises the need to change the culture of consultants as well as to regulate the public–private boundary more effectively. It has the advantage of simplicity, but may be unrealistic. An approach based on rewarding specialists' overall level of commitment to the NHS, their performance against criteria of quality and productivity, and steps to avoid detriment to public patients through the maintenance of private practice, would appear to be more consistent with the values of the UK medical profession.

Another approach might be to raise the incomes of those specialists in fields with extensive private practice opportunities who are committed to working exclusively in the NHS for periods of time, either by increasing their salaries or by paying them supplements for negotiated, additional NHS work. Again, there would need to be monitoring to ensure that the specialists were performing adequately in their salaried, 'core' time. Maynard and Bloor[23] propose a new consultant contract involving a basic salary, supplemented by bonuses and fees for particular items of service, which could be used to reward greater numbers of treatments in fields where private practice opportunities are extensive.

A final aspect of the control and more formal separation of public and private practice to protect equity of access in the NHS relates to patients who move between the public and private sectors during a single treatment episode in order to derive overall advantage from both. For example, it is possible to obtain an early private outpatient assessment for suspected cancer, thereby securing preferential referral into the NHS for subsequent radiotherapy. This source of inequity could be prevented by suitable regulation.

All the above elements of the current arrangements for managing elective services require attention if access is to be improved and made more equitable. Without extensive reform of current relationships between public and private sectors, there is a risk that additional funding for improving surgical waiting times will be lost in the complex series of individually managed waiting 'pools'.

Improve access by making better use of private sector provision

In addition to putting in additional funding for elective treatment, the Government also supports the principle that NHS purchasers should be encouraged to make greater use of the private sector where it can expand capacity unavailable in the NHS or provide services more cost-effectively than the NHS. There has been a particular focus on developments such as private sector diagnostic and treatment centres aimed at providing same-day testing and diagnosis, or specialising in performing high volumes of a limited range of elective procedures. The Institute for Public Policy Research (IPPR) Commission on Public Private Partnerships[24] concluded that a range of public, private and partnership bids should be explored on a pragmatic, case-by-case basis by primary care groups/trusts and health authorities, so that there would be a degree of contestability in the provision of intermediate care, diagnostic and surgical services, with the focus on relative quality and value for money. While the IPPR report correctly highlighted the importance of rigorous prospective assessment of ventures and a focus on transparency (e.g. information disclosure) and performance assessment, it did not explicitly comment on the fact that non-NHS surgical services are mainly provided by NHS staff. As a result, it would be prudent to mitigate the current perverse incentives described above before concluding that the NHS cannot increase its own capacity and productivity in the field of elective surgery and needs to embark on ambitious private and partnership developments.

Better information to monitor quality and equity

In Chapter 7, we noted that it is impossible to compile complete information on the pattern of work of consultants and their quality across both public and private sectors. Performance information on public and private services and providers (both individual specialists and institutions) should be made far more available to the public, in easily accessible forms, as a matter of routine. This is particularly important in the wake of the Bristol Royal Infirmary and other cases, and with the increasing use of private hospitals by the NHS following the Concordat. For example, referring GPs and their patients should be able to find out which departments and possibly, in some cases, which individual consultants have unacceptably high readmission rates for surgical complications before another surgical scandal arises.

Where the public and private sectors provide the same services, it would be a breakthrough to be able to compare local performance routinely rather than having to rely on *ad hoc* research. Such comparisons would be analogous to the comparative reports on the performance of different health plans, their constituent physician groups and the hospitals they use, which are published in parts of the USA. For example, the California Co-operative Healthcare Reporting Initiative is the product of a voluntary collaboration between health care purchasers, health plans and providers in the State. It publishes reports on the relative performance of health plans on clinical measures such as childhood immunisation coverage, as well as consumer responsiveness measures such as speed of receiving care and of claims processing. Similarly, we recommend that private medical insurance policies and premiums charged to different risk groups should be expressed in comparable formats, and that hospitals and specialists be required to state their prices inclusively to allow informed shopping around by patients. Without all these types of information, it will be impossible to see whether current efforts to improve equity within both the public and private sectors and across the two sectors are succeeding.

Conclusions

It would be possible to implement our proposals on equity of financing, coverage and access without creating a large superstructure of law and regulation such as is found, of necessity, in the Netherlands' health care system. The Netherlands is able to pursue the policy goals of a single, equitable, national health insurance scheme even though social and private insurance co-exist. Indeed, the Dutch periodically debate whether their complex public–private arrangements are worth maintaining, or whether they should simply universalise their social insurance scheme, currently confined to lower-income groups. We are, though, proposing that equity and consumer protection criteria should play a far more important role in guiding health services' policy-making from now on. There will need to be some regulatory change to implement our recommendations.

The UK health system is inconsistent in its ability to deliver equity of financing, coverage and access – just as it is variable in its protection and promotion of consumer interests. In spite of recent legislation, the public and private sectors are largely regulated as two separate entities, and their effects on one another are still largely neglected. Yet as the WHO framework for assessing the performance of health care systems makes plain, governments have a responsibility to assure the minimum quality and degree of fairness of all health care, both public and private. At the same time, governments in the UK will have to decide what differences in coverage and access are publicly acceptable between and within the two sectors. That is, they will have to decide how equitable the UK health care system should be and how much public money it is worth spending to bring this about in light of other demands on public resources.

Our recommendations are for a common patient-centred framework to encourage quality and equity of service across both public and private sectors. We believe that that this is a logical extension of the Government's NHS Plan. It is also consistent with the WHO principle that states should take as much responsibility for the fairness of financing, equity of access and quality of health care received by their populations in the private sector as in the public sector.

References

1   World Health Organisation. *The World Health Report 2000*. Geneva: WHO, 2000.

2   Daniels N, Light D, Caplan R. *Benchmarks of Fairness for Health Care Reform*. New York: Oxford University Press, 1996.

3   Commission on Public Private Partnerships. *Building Better Partnerships*. London: IPPR, 2001.

4   Ibid.: 273.

5   National Institute for Clinical Excellence. *Guidance on the Use of Cyclo-oxygenase (Cox) II Inhibitors, Celecoxib, Rofecoxib, Meloxicam and Etodolac for Osteoarthritis and Rheumatoid Arthritis. Technology Appraisal Guidance 27*. London: NICE, 2001.

6   Public Inquiry into Children's Heart Surgery at the Bristol Royal Infirmary 1984–1995. *Learning from Bristol*. Cm 5207. London: Stationery Office, 2001.

7   Rosenau P V. The strengths and weaknesses of public/private partnerships. *American Behavioral Scientist* 2000; 43: 10–34.

8   Green D. Stakeholder health insurance: empowering the poorest patients. *BMJ* 2001; 322: 786–9.

9   Judge K, Benzeval M, Whitehead M, editors. *Tackling Inequalities in Health: an agenda for action*. London: King's Fund, 1995.

10   Acheson D. *Independent Inquiry into Inequalities in Health*. London: Stationery Office, 1999.

11   Tuohy C. *Accidental Logics*. New York: Oxford University Press, 1999.

12   Industry Commission of the Commonwealth of Australia. *Private Health Insurance*. Report No. 57. Canberra: Productivity Commission, 1997.

13   Klein R. Economic and political costs of the NHS: a changing balance sheet? In: Macpherson G, editor. *Our NHS: a celebration of 50 years*. London: BMJ Books, 1998: 106–11.

14   Matthews R. Contributory schemes in theory and in practice. *The Subscriber* 1935; 1: 11–19 and 31.

15   Daniels N, Light D, Caplan R. *Benchmarks of Fairness for Health Care Reform*. New York: Oxford University Press, 1996.

16   Chalkley M, Robinson R. *Theory and Evidence on Cost Sharing in Health Care: an economic perspective*. London: Office of Health Economics, 1997.

17   Light D W. The two-tier syndrome behind waiting lists. *BMJ* 2000; 320: 1349.

18   Daniels N, Light D, Caplan R. *Benchmarks of Fairness for Health Care Reform*. New York: Oxford University Press, 1996.

19   Audit Commission. *The Doctors' Tale*. London: Stationery Office, 1995.

20   Audit Commission. *The Doctors' Tale Continued: the audits of hospital medical staffing*. London: Stationery Office, 1996.

21 Harley M, Jayes B, Yates J. *Long and Short Waiting Times in ENT: a report commissioned by the Department of Health*. Birmingham: University of Birmingham, Inter-Authority Comparisons and Consultancy, 1999.

22 Hefford B, Holmes A. Booking systems for elective services: the New Zealand experience. *Australian Health Review* 1999; 22: 61–73.

23 Maynard A, Bloor K. Reforming the contract of UK consultants. *BMJ* 2001; 322: 541–4.

24 Commission on Public Private Partnerships. *Building Better Partnerships*. London: IPPR, 2001.